ONCOLOGY SOCIAL WORK

A Clinician's Guide

D1551318

DANNETTE HARTZ
Social Work
2080.

ONCOLOGY SOCIAL WORK

A Clinician's Guide

Naomi M. Stearns, MSW
Marie M. Lauria, MSW
Joan F. Hermann, MSW
Paula R. Fogelberg, MSW

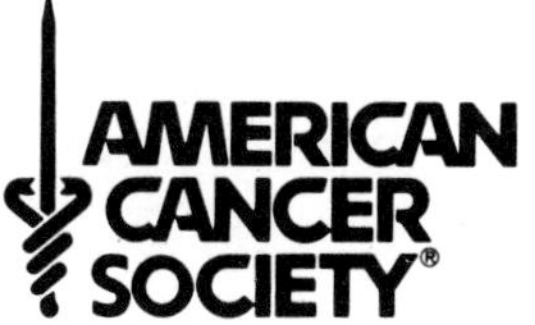

The American Cancer Society, Inc., Atlanta, GA 30329

(c) 1993 by the American Cancer Society.
All rights reserved.
Published 1993. First edition 1993
Printed in the United States of America

97 96 95 94 5 4 3 2 1

Library of Congress Cataloging-in-Publication Data

Oncology social work : a clinician's guide / [edited by] Naomi M. Stearns ... [et al.].
p. cm.
Includes bibliographical references and index.
ISBN 0-944235-08-5
1. Medical social work. 2. Cancer--Patients--Counseling of. 3. Cancer. I. Stearns, Naomi M.
[DNLM: 1. Neoplasms--psychology. 2. Social Work. 3. Sociology, Medical. QZ 200 058255 1993]
HV687.048 1993
362. 1 ' 96994--dc20
DNLM/DLC
for Library of Congress 92-48370
CIP

CONTENTS

PART 3: CANCER IN CHILDREN

PART 4: PROFESSIONAL ISSUES

PART 5: RESOURCES

PART 6: APPENDICES

FOREWORD

The social worker plays a key role in the fight against cancer. In recognition of the vital importance of that role, the American Cancer Society asked social workers from throughout the United States to construct and contribute to a text that could serve as a resource both for social workers without oncolocy training as well as new oncology social workers entering the field. The editors, who are leading American Cancer Society volunteers, collaborated to develop the concept for this text and then to recruit foremost authorities to contribute chapters to the book. The result of this effort is the first edition of *Oncology Social Work: A Clinician's Guide.*

It is our hope that every social worker whose practice includes cancer patients and their families–both social workers speicalizing in oncology as well as general practice social workers–will find this book a valuable resource.

We would like to express our appreciation to the authors and editors who so generously volunteered their time and expertise to produce this text. It is our belief that their many hours spent in researching and writing will ultimately contribute to the quality of care delivered to patients and families dealing with cancer.

–Gerald P. Murphy, MD
Chief Medical Officer
American Cancer Society

–Arlene E. Robinovitch, MSW
Director of Patient Services
American Cancer Society

INTRODUCTION

Naomi M. Stearns, MSW, LICSW
Marie Lauria, MSW, ACSW
Joan Hermann, MSW, ACSW
Paula R. Fogelberg, MSW, LCSW

Cancer has profound biopsychosocial effects, and social workers have much to offer toward the successful management of the illness experience. Many medical social workers specialize in oncology, but a greater number see cancer patients and their families as part of their client population. Others, based in community agencies, see a steadily increasing number of cancer patients, their family members, or both in their practices. Whether in hospitals or community-based facilities, social workers in many settings face challenges in working with cancer patients. Just as the medical management of cancer is highly specialized, social work encompasses a body of knowledge and skills applicable to families facing cancer. This text presents information about cancer diagnosis and treatment, the ways pediatric and adult patients and their families experience cancer, the range of social work interventions applied in cancer care, professional issues in oncology social work, and the identification and access of available resources. This resource book is not intended to be the definitive oncology social work text but instead, it is meant to provide an overview of the field. It is our hope that it will provide the reader with a foundation on which to begin oncology practice and serve as a useful reference as experience grows.

Oncology social work is a dynamic field with a strong theoretical and practical history. Over the years there has been a gradual shift in focus from a speciality that dealt almost exclusively with terminal illness and chronicity to one of coping with treatment and its side effects and adapting to long-term survival. Regardless of the prognosis of the patient, social workers have much to contribute. The crisis intervention skills of social workers lend themselves to managing the predictable and characteristic crisis points. These skills can be well used as families learn how to live within the demands of a chronic illness. Social workers are also skillful in mobilizing the team of healthcare professionals called upon to deliver comprehensive cancer care. While all members of the cancer care team should be equipped to provide basic support to patients and their families, social workers are particularly skilled in helping patients and families with behavioral and psychodynamic issues. Changes in health care resources and reimbursement patterns have increased the emphasis on the social worker's discharge planning expertise. Given the chronic and complex nature of cancer, social workers interested in oncology have the opportunity for a multifaceted, rich practice using the entire repertoire of professional skills.

Oncology social work offers tremendous rewards, primarily the opportunity to make a substantive, qualitative difference in the quality of patient and family life. Social workers new to the field are often surprised to observe the way patients and their families manage to deal with the stresses of the illness. The opportunity to share in the patient's struggle and potential mastery of problems provides tremendous satisfaction for helping professionals. Oncologic practice provides an opportunity for long-term, intense relationships with patients and families. For social workers, whose professional effectiveness depends upon the quality of relationships, the power of these connections can be quite compelling. This work also generates a process of self-discovery and growth. Cancer challenges our philosophy of life, spirituality, and personal and professional value systems. The social work commitment to self-exploration and insight in the service of client growth offers additional benefits to patients and professionals.

For social workers interested in advancing their expertise in oncology, this text may be a first step. More important will be formal education experiences combined with significant patient and family contact, the best teacher for any specialization. The American Cancer Society, in its commitment to the education of health care professionals, offers fellowships in oncology social work at the graduate-student level. Local and national conferences for professionals are also available. Professional literature is a rich source of both medical and psychosocial information. Some hospitals and comprehensive cancer centers also offer intensive courses for beginning and advanced practitioners in psychosocial oncology. The National Association of Oncology Social Workers (NAOSW) offers standards of practice and, as does the Association of Pediatric Oncology Social Workers (APOSW), provides professional education. Information about these opportunities is available in the Resources chapter and appendices of this book.

It is our hope that social workers who are interested in oncology will pursue these opportunities for professional development. Recent advances in cancer treatment have resulted in realistic hope for successful management of the illness. This hopefulness also extends to the quality of patient and family life and mastery of the challenges of cancer. Professional satisfaction will depend upon clinical competence, sensitivity to the human condition, and a belief in people and their capacity to grow. The practice of oncology social work is an opportunity to realize the value and richness of the human experience and of our profession.

CANCER MYTHOLOGY

Joan Hermann, MSW, ACSW

Because of the nature of cancer and its historical association with hopelessness and death, there is a mythology associated with the disease about which social workers should be knowledgeable. Cancer myths are incorrect beliefs and attitudes that interfere with the patients' understanding of his or her particular disease and therefore, his or her ability to manage it most effectively. What we believe about cancer is based on a variety of factors including family history, personal experience with loved ones, education, cultural and religious factors, and emotional responses to the illness. An individual combines these influences and his or her physical symptomatology (or absence of it) with what he or she has heard from medical professionals to construct a perception of the situation. A person's intelligence does not necessarily determine what is believed, especially with a disease that provokes universal fear for most people.

While social workers do not need to possess voluminous or detailed information about cancer before beginning to work with patients, it is important to know the basic facts about an individual's particular cancer and the expected side effects or sequelae of treatment. Patients and their families often do not realize that their beliefs are incorrect or distorted, so the treatment team is not questioned about them. However, these beliefs often surface in a comprehensive psychosocial assessment and it is here that intervention to correct for misinformation can begin. Therefore, social workers should actively assess patients' understanding of their cancer and its treatment in order to influence the accuracy of their information.

Cancer mythology falls into three categories:

1. Questions about the disease itself
2. Questions about treatment
3. Questions about psychosocial adaptation or coping.

QUESTIONS ABOUT CANCER

1. Is cancer contagious?

This is not an easy myth to deal with as people are usually reluctant to acknowledge it as a concern. It can appear foolish to even ask the question so social workers can raise it as "something which some patients worry about." The idea of "catching" cancer from someone else probably developed long ago when little was known about the disease except that most people did not survive. Fears and social stigma resulted in avoidance, the more subtle forms of which can still be a problem today. Social workers should prepare patients for the possibility of changes in their social relationships as a result of a cancer diagnosis. There are ways that patients can reach out to others if they sense an uneasiness or withdrawal of social support. Patients who understand that such behavior is often the result of others' fear and personal vulnerability often deal more easily with it.

2. Are all cancers inherited?

The public does not understand the biological complexity of cancer, so the disease often is conceptualized as being related to a single agent rather than a multiplicity of genetic, familial, and environmental factors. This combines with a universal need to assign meaning to catastrophic events and results in many new cancer patients grappling with the issue of causality. Sometimes the most obvious place to begin this search is within the family. Some people believe that cancer runs in families and if one family member has it, others are likely to develop the disease. It is true that the risk factors for certain types of cancers (breast, colon, and melanoma) tend to be familial. The risk may be increased by other factors such as poor diet, smoking, hormonal influences, or occupational exposure that when combined with a family history of the disease can put certain people at a slightly higher risk of developing a cancer. Social workers can be helpful in guiding these families toward regular screening programs.

However, if the family history includes people with different kinds of cancers (an uncle with lung cancer, a grandparent with leukemia), individual family members are no more likely than the general population to develop a cancer. Likewise, if a person has bladder cancer, prostate cancer, or a brain tumor, their children cannot "inherit" this type of cancer. Occasionally we become aware of "cancer families" in which unusually high numbers of family members have the disease. These families are being intensively studied by the National Cancer Institute but so far, definite conclusions have not been reached about this very small group of people. This phenomenon is still not understood by cancer researchers but in no way is it viewed as proof that cancer is an inherited disease.

It is important for social workers to explore all of the patient's theories about etiology–including the inheritance issues–so that unnecessary feelings of self-blame and guilt do not interfere with coping.

3. CAN CANCER BE CAUSED BY AN INJURY?

Injuries such as bruises, cuts, or broken bones cannot cause cancer. This idea is popular because a person may suffer an injury, see a doctor and, coincidentally, a tumor that has existed for awhile will be discovered. A fall or an injury to the breast cannot cause breast cancer. An athlete with a bruise or swelling in the leg will not develop a bone tumor.

Cancer is a complex disease, arising from a combination of many factors. If there were one single cause of cancer, such as an injury, the cure would have been discovered long ago. An exception to this is lung cancer: certain kinds can be directly linked to smoking. Even with lung cancer, however, there is no one simple cause because not all smokers will develop lung cancer and some people who have never smoked will develop the disease.

4. IS CANCER A DISEASE OF THE ELDERLY?

Many people think they do not have to worry about developing cancer until they are older. However, only about 50% of all cancers occur in people over 65. People under the age of 40 often think they have no chance of getting cancer and delay seeing their doctor if they have a worrisome symptom. Some cancers, like testicular cancer or Hodgkin's disease, are more likely to occur in younger people. For childhood cancers, an estimated 7800 new cases will be diagnosed in 1992 in contrast to 1 130 000 new cases in adults.†

For social workers, it is important to be sensitive to some of the attitudinal problems associated with cancer and age. The elderly may be viewed as less eligible for aggressive curative treatment because of their age and pre-existing medical conditions. Cancer may also be perceived as more consistent with life's natural developmental course, as opposed to cancer in the young which is often viewed as more tragic. Obviously, the elderly are entitled to normal feelings of anger and the emotional turmoil associated with adjusting to a catastrophic event.

5. DOES PERSONALITY OR STRESS CAUSE CANCER?

Some researchers have been interested in the question of the relationship of an individual's personality and the development of cancer. For instance, several studies have concluded that people who have difficulty expressing anger are more likely to develop cancer. These studies have serious flaws in the way they were conducted, and most cancer specialists do not believe any link exists between personality and cancer. Cancer is too complex a disease to be explained by a single cause. There is no scientific evidence that a person's personality could cause cancer to develop.

The same may be said about the idea that people under severe stress are more likely to develop cancer because they were emotionally upset for a long period of time. This area of research, however, deserves further study. There seems to be some association between severe stress, *combined with other physical and genetic factors,* and heart disease, ulcers, and other ailments. This is a complex question but so far, there is no scientific evidence proving that stress can cause cancer. There is also no evidence that cancers will metastasize faster in patients who are emotionally upset or that stress will counteract the anti-tumor effects of treatment.

For some patients the personality issue can become a significant one. Social workers know that "personality" does not change as a result of counseling or a patient's determination, so it is important that patients understand that personality is fairly fixed. However, patients and families can work on developing better ways of dealing with

† *Cancer Facts & Figures -1992. Atlanta, Ga: American Cancer Society.*

stress and it is in that direction that psychosocial intervention is the most fruitful.

6. Is cancer inevitably painful?

The myth that cancer is always painful is associated with people's fear of the disease. Some cancers cause no physical pain. Other patients who die from cancer may experience mild to severe pain. Many people do not realize that more advances have been made in the treatment of pain than in the treatments associated with curing cancer. We can reassure the vast majority of patients with extensive disease that with adequate treatment they can remain comfortable. If patients suffer from severe pain, they or their families must be aggressive in seeking the consultation of a pain specialist.

Another myth is that pain is an early symptom of cancer. This myth is responsible for delays in diagnosis because many people think that if changes in their bodies are not painful there is less cause for concern. However, many cancers in their early stages produce no pain, so people should not wait until something hurts before they see their doctor. Early detection still offers the best opportunity for cure or long-term control.

Social workers new to oncology will become aware that there is a very strong grass roots movement in this country to educate the public and professionals alike about the management of cancer pain. The American Cancer Society, National Cancer Institute, and multiple State Pain Initiatives have been established to counteract the undertreatment of pain and misinformation surrounding the issue. The public and many professionals still worry about issues of addiction, which have repeatedly been disproven in clinical studies. This is only one of many erroneous ideas associated with cancer pain that cause patients and their families unnecessary suffering. It is vitally important that social workers practicing in oncology educate themselves about this problem so they can advocate for patients under their care. Additional information can be obtained from the American Cancer Society, National Cancer Institute, and the Wisconsin Pain Initiative, to name a few. Since social workers typically see more patients with progressive disease, correct information about the pain issue is essential to helping patients achieve optimal management of their symptoms.

7. Does cancer mean certain death?

The association of cancer with inevitable death is changing gradually as survival statistics improve. Today, almost half of all people with newly diagnosed cancers can be cured. Hundreds of thousands of people have already been cured and are leading normal lives. Cancer is truly a chronic disease rather than an inevitably fatal one. People generalize about cancer and think of it as one disease rather than over one hundred different diseases, each with its own unique pattern of development, receptivity to treatment, and prognosis. Some cancers that used to be fatal are curable with the correct treatment (e.g., testicular, certain leukemias, Hodgkin's disease). Other cancers remain very difficult to treat. Patients must understand their particular situations and must understand that questions about prognosis cannot be adequately addressed until the patient's response to the initial treatment is demonstrated. Some patients become fixated on statistics that have meaning for large groups of individuals rather than one person. Many people believe that the uncertainty associated with the question of survival is the most difficult challenge of all. Social work intervention can be most helpful to patients in meeting this challenge.

The myth that cancer equals inevitable death is problematic because patients can be perceived as "dying" rather than "living." Even if cancer recurs after the initial treatment, long-term control of the disease is possible. An ongoing focus on living is essential to a reasonable quality of life. Social workers need to respond aggressively to a client's debilitating helplessness yet remain realistic about pre-existing personality or organic factors that interfere with quality of life.

QUESTIONS ABOUT CANCER TREATMENT

1. Does exposing a tumor to the air during surgery cause cancer to spread?

Before advances in early detection and treatment, surgery often resulted in the discovery of widely metastatic disease from which the patient subsequently died. This led to the belief that surgery either caused cancer or "exposure to the air" resulted in its rapid acceleration. An operation cannot cause a cancer to develop or to spread. Occasionally, surgery can cause a tumor to "seed" (spread) into the incision site. This situation is predictable and is not necessarily a surgical mistake. When such "seeding" is unavoidable, the surgeon often will suggest chemotherapy or radiation to destroy any microscopic cells that may have escaped from the tumor. People may still believe in the myth because a patient often feels much sicker after surgery than before. Although this is due to the normal postoperative recovery process, the surgery becomes the culprit. Fortunately, advances in diagnostic testing have made it possible to know a great deal about a patient's tumor and potential areas of metastases prior to diagnosis. Therefore, there are fewer "exploratory" operations being done today to answer diagnostic questions. Still, the complete removal of a tumor offers the best chance for cure. If a patient is resisting surgery as a treatment option, it is important to explore his or her belief system before settling for a second-best treatment approach. Likewise, a patient who expects curative surgery in the face of metastatic disease will be educated about chemotherapy or radiation therapy or both as better treatment options.

2. DO ALL THE CANCER DRUGS CAUSE THE SAME EFFECTS?

People generalize about chemotherapy and tend to believe that all chemotherapy treatments are alike. There are approximately 40 standard anti-cancer drugs now in use. Each of these drugs has different side effects ranging from very mild ones to severe ones. Chemotherapy works on cells that are dividing. Hair follicle cells, cells in the gastrointestinal area (mouth, stomach, and intestine), and blood cells divide rapidly and therefore are more active than other cells in the body. Consequently, side effects such as hair loss, nausea and vomiting, diarrhea, and changes in blood counts are more common, but still do not affect all patients in the same way.

Regardless of their severity, side effects can be controlled with other medications or with behavioral treatments such as relaxation training. Nausea is a side effect that most cancer patients expect to experience. Not all chemotherapeutic agents cause nausea, but patients taking any that do are given additional drugs to keep nausea under control. Side effects cannot always be totally controlled, but there are many antidotes that will help patients feel as comfortable as possible.

Hair loss is another example. While not all chemotherapy causes hair loss, patients can be informed that when it does, the hair usually grows back.

Physicians can predict those side effects that are most likely to occur for an individual patient. Everyone's body is different–patients may experience hardly any side effects or may experience many of them. However, there is often no way to predict *how* an individual is likely to react before treatment begins. Experiencing or not experiencing side effects has nothing to do with whether the treatment is working.

Social workers can encounter patients whose fears about chemotherapy cause them to reject this therapeutic modality. Chemotherapy can cure certain cancers or can result in better symptom management, so it is important for patients to have a realistic understanding of what to expect. Some patients may have known others who received chemotherapy without adequate management of side effects, so their fears must be addressed prior to starting treatment. Because of the variability and individuality of a patient's response to chemotherapy drugs, it often helps to encourage patients to receive the first course and evaluate their bodies' response to it before making a premature judgment about treatment efficacy or their tolerance to it. This gives patients the benefit of a most-informed choice rather than one based on distorted information.

3. Is radiation therapy dangerous or painful?

As with chemotherapy, people also generalize about radiation therapy, thinking that its side effects are all the same. Radiation therapy is painless, does not cause people to become "radioactive," and is not the therapy of last resort for hopeless cases. Radiation therapy can be curative, as in treating women with certain breast cancers who are candidates for removal of the lump (lumpectomy) rather than the entire breast. The side effects associated with radiation are determined by the area of the body being treated and the amount of radiation given. People do not become sterile from radiation except in certain kinds of treatments to the pelvic area. Today, thanks to modern technology, even this is often avoidable.

The most common side effect associated with radiation is fatigue, especially if treatments last for five or six weeks. This is due to the actual treatment effects combined with the physical and emotional strain of daily visits to the treatment center. As with all cancer treatment, physicians can predict what a patient is most likely to experience. Many patients continue to work throughout their radiation therapy but may need to readjust their schedules or workload temporarily.

Even if radiation therapy cannot cure, it can be extremely effective in symptom management. A typical use of radiation is for bone metastases, which can be painful. As with chemotherapy, social workers can help patients deal with their apprehension about radiation therapy in the interest of their most-informed choices about treatment.

4. IS THE TREATMENT WORSE THAN THE DISEASE?

Some people believe the cancer treatment is worse than the disease itself. This is a particularly dangerous idea because an untreated cancer is far more dangerous than a cancer that is being treated. If a tumor is left to grow untreated, it will eventually interfere with body functions and be more difficult to manage. Treatment can be curative, meaning aggressive enough to eliminate the cancer, or palliative, meaning to control the symptoms of the illness, prolong a patient's life or both. Palliative treatment used to control symptoms (for example, radiation to manage spinal cord compression) often results in a better quality of life for a longer time.

People with advanced cancer often question how long to continue with treatment. Patients and families need information from their physicians in order to adequately assess treatment benefits and risks. Professional staff often grapple with identical questions about the impact of continued treatment on a patient's quality of life. The answers to these dilemmas ultimately depend on the physical and psychosocial needs of the patient and family. Some patients may seem to terminate treatment too quickly while others may need to continue in the absence of any obvious benefit. While it can be extremely difficult for staff to support what we perceive to be a misguided choice,it is probably best to err on the side of what a patient believes to be in his or her best interest.

QUESTIONS ABOUT HOW TO COPE WITH CANCER

1. DO PEOPLE REALLY WANT TO KNOW IF THEY HAVE CANCER?

Not so long ago, the question of whether to disclose a cancer diagnosis was a real issue for physicians, patients, and families. Few effective curative treatments were available. It was thought that patients would become hopelessly depressed or even suicidal if they knew the true nature of their disease. Fortunately, with what we now know about cancer therapies and human psychology disclosure is no longer a clinical issue in a modern treatment setting. Studies have shown that the overwhelming majority of patients want and need to know their diagnosis. It is unethical to withhold such information and still adhere to the principles of informed consent and patient self-determination. In addition to the ethical and psychological issues, cancer is an impossible secret to keep.

Health professionals will still encounter people who ask that patients be shielded from knowing they have cancer. Most clinicians understand this attempt to "protect" the patient as a phenomenon associated with complex family dynamics and the power of the feelings associated with cancer. Family members who request such secrecy need help in dealing with their own overwhelming reactions. They must be able to separate their feelings from what the patient needs in order to cope with the situation most effectively. People do not come into this world knowing how to deal with cancer; they only learn through the experience. The treatment team need to share the positive benefit of their experience with cancer disclosure so that the family has the benefit of that knowledge. Equally important is the family's ability to develop trust in the physician to deliver information in a sensitive, truthful, and enabling way. Information, much like medication, needs to be titrated so that patients will receive what they want and need. This will vary from one individual to another, but the ability to individualize our patients' needs is the key to successful interaction with them. Social workers can be enormously helpful in assessing and intervening with patients and their families to ensure their understanding of the diagnosis and their ability to make the most informed choices about treatment options.

2. If patients know their diagnosis, will they become depressed and feel hopeless?

Contrary to what some people think, people with cancer who are informed of their diagnosis and treatment do not become hopelessly depressed. The most important issue is how the information is conveyed from physician to patient. Assuming that the physician communicates with realistic hope, most patients will mobilize themselves after their diagnosis, begin their treatment, and go on with their lives.

Immediately following a diagnosis of cancer, many patients experience a mourning or grieving process that mimics depression. People mourn for the loss of their idea of themselves as healthy and for the loss of certainty and predictability in their lives. This is usually a short-lived phenomenon and is a natural reaction to learning of a potentially life-threatening illness. If mourning continues for several months after treatment ends, counseling may be indicated. At times, however, patients develop depression in response to the diagnosis, or a long-standing depression may be present. Depression is a complex clinical problem and there is significant controversy within the psychosocial oncology field as to its management. Some resist the use of psychotropic medications with the belief that their use will blunt the individual's normal adjustment reaction to a catastrophic event. Others feel strongly that the judicious use of the correct medication can be a powerful tool in assisting adaptation. Depression can be seriously under- or overtreated, depending on the setting and philosophies of the treatment team. The use of psychotropic medications with cancer patients is a complex issue. The disease itself or its treatment can produce organic changes that affect a patient's mood. For this reason, psychiatrists with experience in oncology are the best resources in evaluating and recommending psychotropic therapy. Oncology social workers are often the first to identify patients whose emotional responses are atypical of the normal course of adjustment. For this reason, social workers need to be knowledgeable in this area in order to offer their best clinical service.

3. Is cancer a punishment?

Many patients have a theory about why they have developed cancer, especially when physicians cannot say with certainty what caused the illness. Some patients decide that the diagnosis is a form of punishment for something they have done or not done in the past. Mothers of pediatric cancer patients are particularly vulnerable and often review their pregnancies in an attempt to identify what might have caused childhood cancer. Behind the question of "Why me?" is often the notion that finding the "reason" for the diagnosis will somehow change things. This is not necessarily logical or rational; it merely reflects the way the human mind works. The search for cancer's cause is a natural phenomenon associated with a new diagnosis. Patients often move away from this search as they begin treatment and start to feel more in control. However, personality and family dynamics often complicate the process. A person's self-image and innate sense of optimism or fatalism about life will obviously be influential. The situation becomes even more complex if a patient's behavior has had an effect on the development of cancer, such as smoking and lung cancer, or prolonged sun exposure and melanoma.

This is a rich area for social work intervention. Patients who continue to grapple with self-blame and guilt will have less emotional energy to devote to treatment and successful coping. Regardless of any true association between behavior and a cancer diagnosis, the task for the patient involves forgiveness and acknowledging the lack of predictability and "fairness" in life. Social workers are often the only members of the treatment team to discover a patient's theories about punishment and guilt feelings, so it is important that these theories be explored during the psychosocial assessment.

4. Will a positive attitude influence survival?

The mind/body interplay is not well understood in today's scientific approach to cancer diagnosis and treatment. It is, however, an area of sometimes raging controversy as so called "pop psychology" interacts with behavioral researchers struggling to design credible studies to answer the questions. Most clinicians have anecdotal experience with patients who accomplish much or live longer in spite of overwhelming disease. Regardless of the academic argument, patients and their families often will struggle with the mind over matter dilemma, which takes the form of the relationship between positive attitude or will to live and cancer survival. Most patients are realistic about how they might influence their disease but do realize that a positive attitude will help them feel better and more in control. To this end the behavioral therapist, with the use of techniques such as relaxation and positive imagery, can be very helpful to patients.

One problematic offshoot of the focus on a positive attitude can be a reluctance to allow feelings of sadness, anger, and fear that are appropriate to what patients might be experiencing. Patients may be admonished by others that they "will never get better if you don't stop feeling that way." What is not understood is that feelings that are not dealt with are repressed and can seriously interfere with the building of hope and positive coping strategies.

The other potential difficulty is self-blame if disease recurs. Patients often experience recurrence as a more difficult psychological challenge because of its assault to their defenses, so this obviously requires intervention. Patients and their families need to know that science has not established a definitive connection between cancer survival and attitude, but in a way that does not interfere with their human and necessary desire to exert some control over their lives.

It is all too easy for professionals to assume the extremes of the argument as we grapple with our own feelings of helplessness and identification with our patients. Until research is able to provide more certainty in this complex area, we need to respect our patients' choices about what they find helpful. Obviously, we should not reinforce the notion that the mind can guarantee survival. As clinicians, however, we know that hope for the future and a positive orientation to life will have a profound impact on the quality of our patients' lives. The ability to make a difference in a family's quality of life is the challenge and joy of oncology social work.

CONCLUSION

This chapter has reviewed some of the most common myths associated with cancer. Readers will undoubtedly come upon other incorrect beliefs and attitudes about cancer, the more problematic of which interfere with treatment and effective coping.

Education about cancer is a complex process considering the emotions associated with the disease and its management. Social work skills in dealing with underlying feelings and dynamics will greatly enrich this process. The result will be a better-informed patient able to make more knowledgeable and psychologically sound decisions.

THE NATURE OF ADULT CANCER: MEDICAL DIAGNOSIS AND TREATMENT

David S. Rosenthal, MD

Cancer is not one disease state but rather many, all characterized by the presence of an uncontrolled (i.e., malignant) proliferation of a certain cell in the body. There are numerous types of cells, so there are many types of cancer. In the adult, cells that become malignant most frequently originate in the lung, colon, rectum, breast, skin, or prostate. This chapter will deal with the incidence of cancer, the risk factors associated with some of the common types of adult cancer, the procedures of medical diagnosis and staging, the modalities of therapy, survival statistics, and the late effects of therapy.

It is increasingly necessary to approach treatment of the cancer patient with all available medical and technological resources. The interdisciplinary approach to case management involves the participation of all members of the health-care professional team, including the primary care physician, the oncology specialist, the nurse, the pharmacist, the nutritionist, the clergy, and others. The oncology social worker is a vital member of the team and must be aware of the many implications of the specific diagnoses, therapeutic approaches, and epidemiologic features of the disease.

INCIDENCE

Almost every family will have at least one member in each generation become ill with cancer. The incidence of cancer increases with age and is second only to cardiovascular disease as a major cause of disease-related death in the United States. More than 1 million new cases of cancer are diagnosed each year. Figure 1 shows the age-adjusted cancer death rates for the most frequent forms of cancer noted between the years 1930 and 1988 for men and women.

Several important observations can be made from these data, most notably the rising incidence of deaths due to lung cancer. Today, lung cancer is the leading cause of cancer death in women, surpassing even breast cancer. Of the almost 500 000 deaths due to cancer in the United States each year,[1] tobacco use appears to be the single major factor related to environment or life-style.[2] Of interest is the decreased incidence of deaths due to stomach cancer (Fig. 1). This decline has occurred in both sexes and may be related to improved dietary practices.[3] Overall death rates due to uterine and cervical cancer have also decreased, which may be attributed to better surveillance and the initiation of routine cytological examination (Pap smear) among women.[4] The most common cancer other than skin cancer that affects both men and women over the age of 50 is cancer of the colon and rectum, accounting for an estimated 157 500 new cases in 1991.[1] In children and young adults, cancer is rare; approximately 7 800 cases were diagnosed in 1991 in the United States. It is still the second-leading cause of death in children under the age of 14, accounting for 11% of total deaths in this age group, with accidents being first.[5] The major cancers in the pediatric population are leukemias, lymphomas, and brain tumors. In young adults, testicular tumors, ovarian malignancies, lymphomas, and leukemias are the most common forms of cancer.[6]

EPIDEMIOLOGY AND ETIOLOGY

What makes a normal cell become malignant? What makes an oncogene turn itself on within a cell? These and similar questions have been the subject of intensive investigation throughout the past decade. It has been well recognized in animals that viruses, radiation, and/or chemicals can increase the incidence of cancer in an experimental setting.[7] In humans, viruses play a small role in cancer causation.[8] The Epstein-Barr virus (EBV) has been implicated in lymphomas and nasopharyngeal carcinoma, while the hepatitis B virus is associated with liver cancer.[9] More recently, herpes and human papilloma viruses (HPV) have been associated with an increased incidence of cancer of the cervix.[10] In the 1980s, a new class of viruses, human T cell lymphotropic viruses (HTLV),was linked to a type of acute lymphocytic leukemia.[11] Also, this group of viruses includes the human immunodeficiency virus (HIV) that is the cause of acquired immunodeficiency syndrome (AIDS). Although AIDS is a virally transmitted disease, many AIDS patients will develop cancers such as

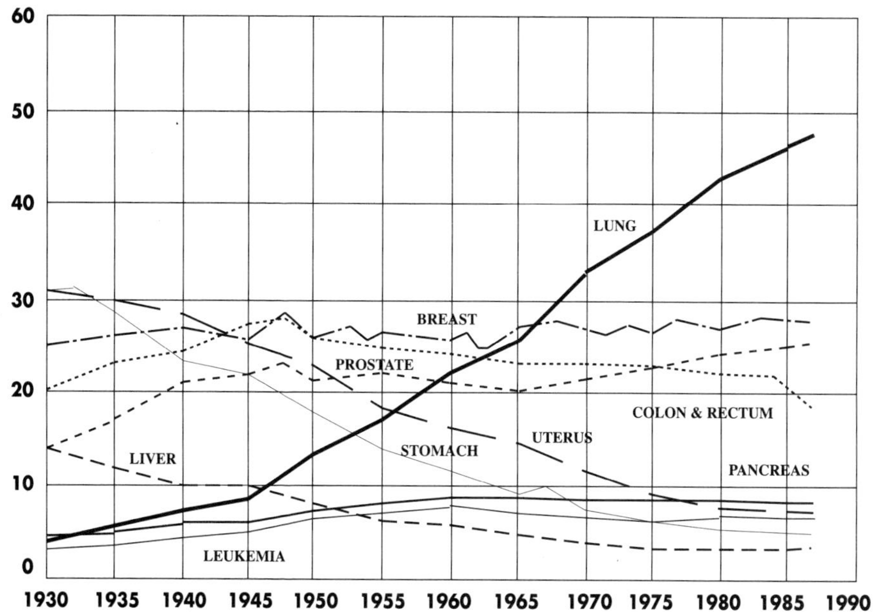

Figure 1. Age-adjusted cancer death rates by site, United States, 1930-1988. Rate for the population is standardized for age on the 1970 US population. Rates are for both sexes combined except breast and uterus (female population only) and prostate (male population only). Sources of data: National Center for Health Statistics and Bureau of the Census, United States. Reprinted from Cancer Facts and Figures 1992.[1]

Kaposi's sarcoma and lymphomas. Irradiation as an etiologic agent in cancer has been the subject of much controversy. Although high levels of radiation, as is used in the treatment of Hodgkin's disease, can increase the incidence of leukemia in that specific population,[12] low levels of radiation have not been proven to cause leukemias or lymphomas. Ultraviolet light (UVL) and excessive sun exposure are definite risk factors for skin cancers such as basal cell carcinoma and melanoma.[13] In cancer epidemiology, occupational medicine has emerged as an important field with major investigations into exposure to toxins, chemicals, and radiation. It has been demonstrated, for instance, that contact with asbestos and polycyclic hydrocarbons may result in lung cancer, while exposure to vinyl chloride and benzene have been linked to liver cancer and acute myelogenous leukemia (AML), respectively.[14]

There is increasing evidence that nutrition plays a role in many cancers. High-fat diets are associated with a higher risk of colon, breast, endometrial, and prostate cancers.[14] A low-fat, high-fiber diet appears to offer some protective effect against bowel cancer. The incidence of gastric cancer in native Japanese populations is high compared to other countries, although the incidence decreases in that population upon migration to the United States. Excessive alcohol consumption has been linked with liver cancer and increases the incidence of other cancers when accompanied by tobacco use.[14] Nasopharyngeal, oral, esophageal, and gastric cancers are increased in incidence secondary to alcohol consumption and tobacco use.

Epidemiologic evidence has shown that many cancers occur at an increased rate among families. For example, the chance of developing breast cancer is higher in a woman whose mother or sister has had the disease. The revolution in our potential to study genetic makeup has revealed that many cancers begin with genetic defects that may be passed on from generation to generation. Certain illnesses or conditions may predispose an individual to a higher risk of cancer, as in patients with a long history of untreated, active ulcerative colitis. Such patients have a higher incidence of colon cancer. In many cases, it is a combination of these factors that result in cancer, as in patients with familial polyposis. Familial polyposis is a condition that runs in families and is genetically determined. It causes the development of multiple benign polyps. These polyps frequently transform to cancer, sometime as early as the teenage years, so careful follow up is required in these patients. Clearly, all health care providers should be aware of patients' family histories and the potential effect this information has on cancer risk.

Certain cancers predispose to further cancers; for example, many women with a particular type of breast cancer–lobular carcinoma in situ–develop a primary cancer in another site within the same breast or in the opposite breast.[15] Some cancer therapies have been implicated, as well, in the development of a second cancer.[16]

The good news is that, as we learn more about sources of cancer, we are gaining insight into how some cancers can be prevented (Table 1). Also, some cancers that are otherwise potentially deadly can be treated with great success *if detected early.* Early detection measures are available for several cancers (Table 2) and much work is being done to develop and test new and more sensitive methods. These factors–early detection and prevention–will be the impetus for cancer control in the coming decades. For this reason, health education will be increasingly important in every cancer control effort.

The American Cancer Society has made a major contribution to cancer control by developing guidelines for routine checkups for asymptomatic individuals. The guidelines are aimed at detecting the disease at an early, potentially curable stage. Table 3 summarizes the American Cancer Society guidelines. It has been estimated that, if these guidelines were followed, more than one-half of cancer cases and/or deaths seen today might be prevented.[14]

ESTABLISHING THE DIAGNOSIS

Although cancer may be suspected on the basis of a patient's symptoms, history, and physical examination, a diagnosis can only be confirmed on the basis of a tissue biopsy and pathologic study of the specimen removed. The accurate diagnosis of the cell of origin and staging of the malignancy require a sufficient amount of tissue. This can be accomplished by removing the entire tumor (excisional biopsy) or a piece of the mass (incisional biopsy). A needle aspiration is a less invasive procedure that can be used when a suspicious mass is seen on mammography or palpated in the breast. Fine needle aspirations may be helpful in the initial evaluation of a lung mass seen on chest x-ray, or an abdominal mass seen on CT scan or ultrasound. A needle guided by CT scan can be inserted into a mass in the pancreas, for example, thereby avoiding major surgery and general anaesthesia. Aspirations may yield small amounts of tissue, insufficient for diagnosis.

Once obtained, all tissue specimens are analyzed by microscopy, but further investigative studies such as electron microscopy, immunologic studies, and in some cases chromosomal and gene analysis may be required. The role of the pathologist is to confirm the cancer diagnosis, differentiating it from disorders masquerading as malignancies such as infections or benign tumors. Following confirmation, the next step is to determine the cell of origin. Although routine methods of examination may be adequate, frequently the tissue does not resemble any normal tissue and requires histochemistry, cell receptor studies, and immunologic and/or cytogenetic study to determine the origin. Undifferentiated malignancies challenge the pathologist, who requires sufficient biopsy

Table 1

SOME KNOWN (K) OR PROPOSED (P) SOURCES OF CERTAIN CANCERS AND MEASURES TO PREVENT THEM*

SOURCE	CANCER	PREVENTION MEASURES
Smoking	Lung (K) Bladder (K) Esophageal (K)	Don't start smoking Stop smoking
Chewing tobacco, snuff	Oral (K)	Don't use tobacco products
Sun exposure	Skin cancers (K) Melanoma (K)	Use protective clothing and sunscreen with SPF >15 Avoid exposure when radiation is most intense; protect from reflected light (snow, water, etc.)
Alcohol†	Head & neck (K) Oral (K)	Use moderately, if at all
Occupational exposure		
Asbestos Benzene	Lung (K) Bladder (P) Acute Myelogenous leukemia (K)	Avoid exposure and use proper protection if available
High dietary fat	Breast (P) Colorectal (P)	Follow the American Cancer Society's Nutrition Guidelines

* *Proposed means that early evidence of association has been shown in one or more studies and that further studies are in progress.*

† *Especially in combination with smoking, which greatly increases risk.*

Table 2
EARLY DETECTION TECHNIQUES

For colorectal cancer
- Fecal blood test
- Digital rectal examination
- Sigmoidoscopy
- Barium enema
- Flexible colonoscopy

For cervical cancer
- Pap test

For breast cancer
- Breast self-examination
- Physical examination
- Mammography

For prostate cancer
- Digital rectal examination

For skin cancer
- Total skin examination

Table 3

SUMMARY OF AMERICAN CANCER SOCIETY RECOMMENDATIONS FOR THE EARLY DETECTION OF CANCER IN ASYMPTOMATIC PEOPLE

		Population	
TEST OR PROCEDURE	**SEX**	**AGE**	**FREQUENCY**
Sigmoidoscopy	M&F	50 & over	Every 3 to 5 years based on advice of physician
Stool guaiac slide test	M&F	Over 50	Every year
Digital rectal examination	M&F	Over 40	Every year
Pap test	F	All women who are or who have been sexually active, or have reached age 18, should have an annual Pap test and pelvic examination. After a woman has had three or more consecutive satisfactory normal annual examinations, the Pap test may be performed less frequently at the discretion of her physician.	
Pelvic examination	F	18-40	Every 1-3 years with Pap test
		Over 40	Every year
Endometrial tissue sample	F	At menopause, women at high risk*	At menopause
Breast self-examination	F	20 and older	Every month
Breast clinical examination	F	20-40	Every 3 years
		Over 40	Every year
Mammography†	F	40-49	Every 1-2 years
		50 & over	Every year
Health counseling and	M&F	Over 20	Every 3 years
cancer checkup††	M&F	Over 40	Every year

* *History of infertility, obesity, failure to ovulate, abnormal uterine bleeding, or estrogen therapy.*

† *Screening mammography should begin by age 40.*

†† *To include examination for cancers of the thyroid, testicles, prostrate, ovaries, lymph nodes, oral region, and skin.*

(Source: American Cancer Society. *CA: A Journal for Clinicians.* 1992; 42:45.)

material to perform the additional analyses.

The pathologist also "grades" the cancer according to the tumor's virulence or rapidity of growth. Grade is a determinant of prognosis. In addition, the microscopy studies will determine whether the surgical excision was complete. For example, after the surgeon removes a localized cancer of the bowel, it is important to know if the resected margins are free of cancer. Persistent tumor might signify a poor prognosis with both immediate and delayed complications.

After a biopsy the patient often experiences extreme anxiety while awaiting the final results. Although a "quick look" or "frozen section" may differentiate a benign tumor from a cancer, rarely will a pathologist make any final diagnosis on these rapid studies. Generally, it is preferable to have the complete pathology report before discussing the diagnosis with the patient.

STAGING

Three important determinants of prognosis in cancer are the size of the tumor, the number and location of lymph nodes involved, and the presence or absence of distant metastases. For each cancer there are internationally recognized criteria for staging. Staging is an extremely important component of care of the cancer patient and will determine treatment and prognosis. For example, Hodgkin's disease spreads in a very orderly fashion. Knowing how far the disease has spread at the time of diagnosis makes it possible to treat the known disease as well as the next site of potential involvement. Similarly, with localized breast cancer, the involvement of axillary nodes significantly changes the prognosis, and this will have an impact on treatment options. Staging systems offer little help in some malignancies, however. For example, acute leukemia involves the marrow and peripheral blood. Because it is essentially widespread at the time of diagnosis, staging offers no added prognostic help.

Completion of staging the cancer may require studies in addition to the primary surgery. The staging work-up could include blood studies with various serum markers that are correlated with active disease, such as carcinoembryonic antigen (CEA) in colon cancer, PSA for prostate, and CA 125 for ovarian cancer; radiologic studies, such as CT scans, magnetic resonance imaging scans, and ultrasound; nuclear medicine studies using various radioisotopes that are sensitive for minimal disease; and/or further surgical procedures.

A breast cancer patient, for example, would have been evaluated first by clinical examination and mammography. Regional lymph nodes in the axillary, supraclavicular, and infraclavicular areas would be examined. Clinical examination has a high likelihood of being inaccurate in the estimation of the extent of malignancy; thus, surgical sampling of the axillary nodes may be important. The pathologist would be asked to determine whether the breast cancer cells have estrogen receptors, a finding that is helpful in determining whether hormonal therapy is appropriate. Further staging would involve a bone scan with plane bone radiographs of any suspicious area on the scan. Blood studies should include liver function tests to explore the possibility of metastatic liver disease.

The staging of breast cancer, therefore, requires knowing the size of the primary site in the breast, involvement of regional lymph node sites, presence or absence of estrogen receptors, and the presence of bone marrow involvement or liver function abnormality. With this information, the physician and patient can make an informed decision regarding therapy.

Because of the unique pattern of Hodgkin's disease spread, a patient with this diagnosis may undergo more involved staging studies including CT studies of the entire abdomen and pelvis, nuclear medicine scans, and lymphograms. Also in selected cases, an exploratory laparotomy that includes a splenectomy and biopsies of the liver and abdominal nodes may be required to explore the possibility of spread from above the diaphragm to below it. Staging procedures are important because the stage of disease determines the therapeutic alternatives. The patient must be reassured that the delay is worthwhile for the benefits gained. Obtaining the information before treatment will prevent rash therapeutic decisions.

Once therapy has begun, the abnormal test results will be followed, hopefully toward resolution and return to normal. This might include the return of a CEA blood level to normal, or the return of findings on a bone scan or CT scan back to normal. Many cancers cannot be followed by routine physical examinations because the residual sites of disease after diagnosis may be in areas such as the retroperitoneum (back of the abdomen), the bones, or other "silent" areas of the body. Diagnostic technology to address this problem is under development. Newer imaging techniques, such as magnetic resonance imaging or tumor markers in the serum, may make it possible to closely follow the resolution or the recurrence of a cancer. Because malignant cells carry specific proteins (monoclonal antibodies) on their surfaces that distinguish them from normal cells, combining monoclonal antibodies with a radionuclide material provides a technique of detecting the presence of active disease anywhere in the body.

TREATMENT

Major advances continue to be made in surgery, radiation therapy, and chemotherapy. New therapeutic modalities have also been developed, such as biologic immune modifiers, bone marrow transplantation, and growth factors.

SURGERY

Table 4 lists the types of surgical procedures that are used in cancer treatment. Cancers are sometimes cured by removal of the primary tumor, such as a simple mastectomy, without any further intervention. A radical resection for a localized cancer may also be indicated, for example, in localized prostate cancer, certain types of breast cancer, or head and neck cancer. Palliative surgery is employed when a cancer is incurable by a resection, but removal of the tumor mass may alleviate suffering by removing an obstruction or preventing bleeding. Cytoreductive surgery is the removal of a large tumor mass (debulking), a procedure that may enhance the effectiveness of a second therapeutic modality such as radiation therapy or chemotherapy. Photodynamic therapy employs a combination of drugs and lasers to destroy cancer cells. A drug that concentrates in certain types of cancer cells, but not in healthy cells, is injected into the patient. A laser operating at a specific light wavelength is then directed at the area of the tumor where it selectively destroys the drug-containing cancer cells. This type of therapy may be very effective in some bladder cancers.

Laser surgery involves the use of a laser focused on a specific tumor site to relieve obstruction, aid in further surgical removal, or combine with chemotherapy or radiation therapy. Extreme thermal changes, or cryoablation, may be applied via probes to symptomatic metastatic lesions in the liver or other sites. The surgeon is also involved in staging procedures, second-look procedures, reconstruction, and indirect surgical technology. Second-look surgical procedures are used in evaluating the responses to therapy and are appropriate for diseases such as ovarian cancer.

Reconstructive surgery may be employed after mastectomy, head and neck surgery, or other physically disfiguring procedures to improve appearance or function. Indirect surgical procedures refer to the placement of Hickman lines or portacatheters to provide easy access for infusions of chemotherapy or blood products. Disfiguring or mutilating radical surgical procedures largely have become a thing of the past because of new knowledge about the effectiveness of less radical surgical procedures and the increased efficacy of both radiation therapy and chemotherapy.

Table 4
SURGICAL PROCEDURES IN CANCER TREATMENT

Curative	Laser
Simple	Cryoablation
Radical	Staging
Palliative	Second look
Cytoreductive	Reconstructive
Photodynamic therapy	Indirect

RADIATION THERAPY

Beams of energy produced by orthovoltage and cobalt via linear accelerators target a high-energy electron directly to the malignant tumor. Table 5 lists types of radiation procedures that are used to destroy cancer cells. The newer radiotherapy techniques are less likely to damage skin and are only effective in the direction of the beam. Thus, radiation therapy is applicable for localized tumors in its curative attempt.

In Hodgkin's disease and testicular tumors, localized radiation therapy to the known site of the disease and the next potential site offers extremely high cure rates. The daily protocol for Hodgkin's disease is radiation therapy for 2-5 weeks, until the maximally tolerated dose for that specific site is reached. Radiation therapy may be used alone as the primary therapy, or in conjunction with surgery or chemotherapy. The sensitivity of various types of tumors to specific radiation doses varies.

Table 5
RADIATION THERAPY TECHNIQUES

Curative	Radiation protectors
Palliative	Hyperthermia
Neoadjuvant	Radio-immunotherapy
Combined modality	Radiation resistance genes
Radiation sensitizers	

Lymphoma and leukemia cells are more sensitive to radiation therapy than are the cells of lung or colorectal cancer. An important consideration in radiation therapy is the ability of normal tissues adjacent to the malignant disease to tolerate radiation. In treating lymphomas, for example, the tradeoff between the damaging effect on lymphoma cells and adjacent normal cells is very acceptable. In the treatment of lung cancer, however, the amount of radiation needed to control and eliminate the disease is extremely high, and this causes significant damage to adjacent normal cells. The kidney and liver are also extremely sensitive to radiation and are excluded from most radiation fields.

Curative radiation therapy is possible in Hodgkin's disease; non-Hodgkin's lymphomas; and cancers of the testis, cervix, prostate, and bladder. As with surgery, other forms of radiation therapy can be palliative or used as neoadjuvant therapy. Palliative radiation therapy is used locally to reduce an obstruction that cannot be approached by surgery. In Hodgkin's disease, for example, a mass in the chest may hamper blood flow by obstructing the superior vena cava. Blood is unable to return to the right side of the heart and the patient's arms, neck, and face swell. Focused radiation therapy will alleviate the obstruction and normal blood flow will resume. Neoadjuvant radiation therapy uses less than curative doses to decrease the tumor size; the intent is to improve the potential for local control by surgery and/or chemotherapy. Similarly, combined modality therapy joins chemotherapy with radiation therapy in an attempt to cure. For example, in Hodgkin's disease patients with widespread or advanced-stage disease, chemotherapy would be the treatment of choice. After chemotherapy, radiation therapy to previous sites of bulk disease would ensure a better outcome by potentially preventing recurrence at the sites.

Certain chemical agents are available that will improve tumor responsiveness to radiation therapy and decease normal tissue damage. These agents are referred to as radiation sensitizers and radiation protectors, respectively. Hyperthermia (induced increase in body temperature) is sometimes employed to increase local effectiveness of radiation therapy.

In some cancers, clinical trials combine radiation with immunotherapy to improve specificity of radiation's killing capability. This involves the preparation of a monoclonal antibody against a specific type of cancer cell, which is then linked with a radiation-emitting substance injected into the bloodstream. The radiation-emitting substance will only be released once the monoclonal antibody has attached itself to the cancer cell.

Many tumors that develop resistance to radiation therapy have been associated with the development of radiation-resistant genes. Research is under way to decrease this sensitivity or to alter these resistant genes, allowing radiation to become a more effective treatment modality.

CHEMOTHERAPY

In 1940, chemotherapy drugs first became available to treat cancer. Since then, chemical agents made from plants, bacteria, and other sources have been used to destroy tumors by inhibiting cell division. Chemotherapeutic approaches to cancer treatment are summarized in Table 6. Different drugs work in different parts of the cell life cycle. For example, methotrexate (used as a single agent) can result in a 30% remission rate in childhood acute lymphocytic leukemia (ALL) by acting at a particular phase of DNA synthesis, interfering with synthesis, repair, and cellular replication. Similarly, alkylating agents such as chlorambucil, cyclophosphamide, and nitrogen mustard destroy malignant cells by producing an effect in dividing cells diffusely throughout the body similar to the effects caused by radiation. By combining medicines that work in different phases of the cell cycle, response rates increase dramatically in disease such as childhood ALL, in Hodgkin's disease, and in non-Hodgkin's lymphoma. This combination chemotherapy approach is also employed in a number of other cancers including ovarian carcinoma, testicular tumors, and choriocarcinoma.

Since most chemotherapy drugs follow first-order kinetics (i.e., a fixed percentage of tumor cells are killed with each course of therapy), the larger the cancer, the less effective the chemotherapy. If the tumor burden is first reduced by surgery and/or irradiation, the chemotherapy is more likely to result in potential cure because the chemotherapy will be more effective against a smaller burden of cancer cells. This combined-therapy approach has made it possible to replace the radical amputation of limbs, performed for osteogenic sarcoma, with limb preservation surgery and intensive chemotherapy to eradicate any systemic disease.

The use of chemotherapy prior to any local treatment modality is referred to as neoadjuvant chemotherapy, in which the therapy is aimed at reducing the size of the primary tumor with the intent to cure the disease. Chemotherapy can create local control, followed by subsequent curative surgery and/or radiation therapy. In head and neck cancer, for example, chemotherapy will not be curative but can reduce the extent of the cancer and may significantly improve survival following surgery and/or radiation therapy.

In animal studies, it has been demonstrated that dose intensity can be a critical factor in the outcome of chemotherapy.[17] However, the toxic effects of chemotherapy limit the amount of chemotherapeutic drugs that can be given. In some cases, bone marrow transplantation has facilitated fivefold to twentyfold increases in chemotherapy doses, and these higher doses have effected substantially higher cure rates for some leukemias and lymphomas.

Combined modality therapy refers to the use of serial courses of chemotherapy and radiation therapy to treat the cancer, as in management of certain stages of Hodgkin's disease, or a combination of surgery and radiotherapy and/or chemotherapy, as in the treatment of various solid tumors.

Besides dose-limiting toxicity, another major problem in chemotherapy is the development of drug resistance, which may be acquired during chemotherapy or may be inherent in the patient's physiology. Many cancers can develop multidrug resistance (MDR), which has been associated with increased expression of a gene product. This MDR phenomenon has stimulated much interest in the study of drug-resistant genes. Overcoming MDR is likely to be difficult, but it is expected that using combination chemotherapy and exploring techniques to reduce or inhibit the drug-resistant genes will play a role in doing so. Finally, combining monoclonal antibodies with toxins or chemotherapeutic agents may also be a way to effectively target cancer cells and attain reduced side effects.

Less toxic than chemotherapy, hormonal therapy offers the possibility of significant objective responses in breast and prostate cancer, but is rarely curative. The administration of pharmacologic doses of sex hormones may impair cancer growth. Certain malignant cells are known to have hormone receptors, making the selection of patients for such therapy possible. The presence of the estrogen receptors on breast cancer cells, for example, is correlated with a good response to hormonal therapy. However, non-endocrine tumors (such as colon cancer) that are found to have hormone receptors do not respond to this form of therapy.

It is important to keep in mind that 50 years of chemotherapy is a relatively short period in the long history of cancer. Newer agents and newer techniques of using older agents continue to be developed.

Table 6
CHEMOTHERAPY APPROACHES IN CANCER TREATMENT

Primary
Single agent
Combination
Adjuvant
Neoadjuvant
High dose with marrow transplantation
Combined modality
Hormonal

IMMUNOTHERAPY AND BIOLOGICALS

One of the most exciting advances in the approach to cancer over the past two decades has been the investigational use of immunotherapy such as monoclonal antibodies, immunotoxins, and biological agents such as interferon, interleukin, and growth factors. These are listed in Table 7.

Monoclonal antibodies, as mentioned previously, have been used as diagnostic tools in tumor imaging and as markers for the presence of disease. These antibodies can also be used as anticancer agents when a tumor-specific antigen can be identified. For example, a specific anti-

Table 7
IMMUNOTHERAPY AND BIOLOGICALS*

SUBSTANCE	DEFINITION	APPLICATION
Interferon	Large protein molecules that help activate the body's immune system and also interfere with the growth of viruses†	High rate of complete remission in HCL; promising outcome in CML, renal cell carcinoma, malignant melanoma, some phases of AIDS
Interleukin II	A lymphokine that supports growth differentiation of thymus-derived lymphocytes. Also called T-cell growth factor†	Experimental in advanced and renal cell cancer
Growth factors	Proteins that encourage cells to grow†	Improve bone marrow reserve; prevent marrow suppression due to chemo- or radiation therapy
Growth factor inhibitors	Substances that inhibit the action of growth factors	Experimental
Monoclonal antibodies	Genetically identical molecules used in diagnosis and therapy. The antibodies can be targeted to specific sites in the body and may be mass-produced by hybridoma cells†	Targets recognized therapy to a specific site in cell (Experimental)

Table 7
IMMUNOTHERAPY AND BIOLOGICALS (CONTINUED)

SUBSTANCE	DEFINITION	APPLICATION
Immunotoxins	A hybrid molecule formed by coupling a toxin or a portion of a toxin to an antibody or antigen molecule; the resulting molecule has the specificity of the antibody or antigen and the toxicity of the toxin	

† Source: The National Cancer Institute.
HCL = hairy cell leukemia;
CML = chronic myelogenous leukemia.

gen referred to as common acute lymphocytic leukemia antigen (CALLA) is frequently present on the surfaces of acute lymphocytic leukemia cells. In the test tube, "CALLA positive" leukemic cells can be cleared or destroyed by the CALLA-specific antibody. In addition, monoclonal antibodies can be "hooked up" or conjugated to toxic agents such as chemicals, radioisotopes, or toxins (immunotoxins). In the test tube, this technique has been shown to be highly effective in destroying target cells. Transference of this technology *in vivo* has been disappointing to date, largely because many tumors do not have specific antigens that are not also common to normal cells.

Cytokines are intercellular messenger proteins. Three subtypes of these proteins have been used in cancer research: interleukins, interferons, and other growth factors.

Interleukins (numbered 1-6) transmit messages between leukocytes and are important molecules normally involved in the body's inflammatory response.

Interferons have an antiviral effect and suppress certain tumor cells both *in vitro* and *in vivo*. Most notably, these agents have been responsible for causing a high complete remission rate in hairy cell leukemia. Promising outcomes with interferons also have been reported with chronic myelogenous leukemia, renal cell carcinoma, malignant melanoma, and certain phases of the AIDS illness.

Other growth factors are proteins that can stimulate hematopoietic stem cells to grow, mature, and differentiate. The growth factor granulocyte-macrophage colony stimulating factor (GM-CSF) acts on the most primitive marrow precursors, causing them to proliferate, mature, and differentiate to adult cells. The potential is to improve marrow reserve and prevent marrow suppression due to chemotherapy and/or radiation therapy.

BONE MARROW TRANSPLANTATION

Bone marrow transplantation (BMT), for many years an investigational treatment, is now considered standard therapy for several diseases including some cancers. For a growing number of patients, BMT offers the best possibility for long-term remission. In some situations the purpose of BMT is to replace chemo- or radiation-damaged marrow (the soft, spongy material in the bone cavities that provide red and white blood cells and platelets) with healthy marrow. In other situations, BMT provides disease-free marrow, either from a donor or from the patient after cancer cells have been eradicated. In both situations, the patient's immune system is altered by the procedure. Some of the diseases treated with BMT are leukemia, non-Hodgkin's lymphoma, and Hodgkin's disease. Bone marrow transplants are also used to treat certain solid tumors such as those of the breast and ovary, and germ cell tumors. It has also been used as treatment for other medical problems such as aplastic anemia, severe combined immunodeficiency disease, thalassemia, and Gaucher's disease.

There are three types of bone marrow transplantation: allogeneic, syngeneic, and autologous.

In *allogeneic transplants*, the marrow comes from a person other than the patient. Usually, the donor is a parent or a sibling, but donors other than relatives are sometimes used. The goal is to find the closest marrow match between donor and recipient, which lessens the chance that the donated marrow will attack the recipient's cells. This situation, known as graft-versus-host disease, occurs in nearly one-half of all allogeneic transplants. Graft-versus-host disease may have both chronic and acute effects and requires prophylactic as well as concurrent treatment to control symptoms. This underscores the importance of having as close a match as possible. "Matching" is based on the numbers of human leukocyte antigens (HLA antigens), which are cell-surface proteins found on lymphocytes, that match between donor and recipient. About 30-40% of patients have an HLA-matched sibling or parent; only 10-15% of patients will be able to locate a suitable unrelated match. Once identified, however, donors may ultimately be disqualified for a variety of reasons or, once tested, may decline to donate. Unrelated donors are recruited through the National Donor Marrow Program; the larger the pool of potential donors, the greater the possibility of finding a match.

A *syngeneic transplant* occurs between identical twins, which provides a perfect match.

Researchers are constantly refining the methods for *autologous* bone marrow transplants, in which the patient (in remission) is his or her own donor. With this type of transplantation, HLA matching is not necessary and the risk of graft-versus-host disease is eliminated. Under general anesthesia, approximately one liter of normal bone marrow is harvested from the patient's hip and pelvis. The harvested marrow may then be treated with radiation or chemotherapy to destroy any possible remaining, undetected cancer cells prior to reinfusing it into patients.

Complications from BMT include risk of infection, bleeding, liver problems, and failure of the transplant itself. Certain long-term effects have been noted, such as infertility, development of cataracts, and the possibility of developing secondary tumors as a result of the therapies used prior to transplant. Certain drugs are routinely given post-BMT to reduce the incidence of, or to manage the symptoms of, graft-versus-host disease and other transplant-related medical problems. These medications are costly and may have significant side effects.

The patient's underlying diagnosis, past response to therapy, and general medical condition at the time of evaluation for BMT are taken into account by the transplant team in determining whether BMT is a treatment of choice and, if so, which type is appropriate. An increasing number of medical centers are performing bone marrow transplants, although some centers specialize in treating certain diseases with this technique. Procedures may vary among centers.

Numerous psychosocial issues confront bone marrow transplant patients and their families. Social workers play a key role in helping patients and families understand what the treatment will involve medically, logistically, emotionally, and financially. Anticipating and negotiating lengthy absences from home, pretreatment procedures, medical isolation, and extended follow-up care can require both patients and families to make significant adjustments. Often, social workers are able to bridge the gap between the referring hospital and the transplant center and provide much-needed continuity post-transplant.

Financial arrangements can be complicated. Third-party payers still may consider certain types of transplants as experimental therapy. Generally, donor expenses for allogeneic transplants are not covered by insurance, and the recipient must assume the donor's financial burden. Prior to the initial consultation with the patient, it is important for the health care team and patient accounting department within the hospital to communicate about the potential transplant. The transplant itself can cost over $100 000. Additional costs include transportation to the center where the transplant will be performed, area housing for the family during the procedure, housing for the patient immediately post-transplant, and follow-up care at the center as well as with the local physician.

SUPPORTIVE THERAPY

The health professional dealing with a cancer patient must realize that he or she is not working in a vacuum. Although the primary doctor-patient relationship is central, both patient and physician need strong support from the entire multidisciplinary health professional team: specialists, members of the tumor board of the hospital, nurses, social workers, nutritionists, clergy, pharmacists, physical and occupational therapists, and dentists. At times, home-health and chronic-care professionals may be involved. The supportive therapy team should be formed early in the diagnostic phase and should be available throughout the course of illness rather than only in response to an acute crisis. This kind of preventive approach helps patients and families anticipate and handle treatment-related problems.

LATE EFFECTS OF TREATMENT AND LONG-TERM FOLLOW-UP

Each year there are increasing numbers of survivors of cancer. Aggressive treatment and improved survival have resulted in greater need for attention to the long-term psychosocial and physical effects of cancer treatment. The long-term effects may be medical (e.g., the late occurrence of toxicity) or psychological (e.g., the failure to cope effectively with the disease). Much is known about the immediate physical side effects of the various therapeutic modalities and more is becoming known about their long-term effects. This is becoming clear in the long-term follow-up of children with all types of cancer and of young adults with Hodgkin's disease. Many years after completing therapy, a childhood cancer survivor may have diminished growth or the potential for a second malignancy. Young adults treated with both chemotherapy and radiation therapy for Hodgkin's disease are at a higher risk for developing a second malignancy such as acute non-lymphocytic leukemia or malignant lymphoma of a non-Hodgkin's type. Unfortunately, despite modern methods of blood testing, chronic hepatitis and AIDS have occurred in long-term survivors who received transfusions. Young men aggressively treated with certain chemotherapeutic agents may develop gonadal dysfunction and permanent infertility. Likewise, women may also experience infertility, and the incidence of these side effects increases with age. Children receiving cranial radiation along with systemic chemotherapy are at risk for dyslexia and other learning disabilities.

In addition to the therapy-related late effects, there may be numerous psychosocial effects. Problems with respect to employment, insurability, and ability to get back in the mainstream of life may occur. Both the physical and the psychosocial late effects may require continuing intervention by the supportive therapy team.

CONCLUSION

The cancer patient's need for integrated team care does not end with complete remission of disease or with achievement of 5-year disease-free survival. Health professionals are still in the learning phase of cancer management. It is already clear that long-term routine follow-up, both medical and psychological, is necessary for an optimal outcome. Further research on long-term effects will enable team members to better predict psychosocial outcomes and needs and to offer more effective support to cancer patients and their families.

REFERENCES

1. American Cancer Society. *Cancer Facts and Figures 1992.* Atlanta, Ga: The American Cancer Society; 1992. p.3.

2. Doll R, Peto R. Causes of cancer: quantitative estimates of avoidable

risk of cancer in the United States today. *J Natl Cancer Inst.* 1981; 66:1191.

3. Palmer S, Bakshi K. Public health considerations in reducing cancer risk: interim dietary guidelines. *Semin Oncol.* 1983; 10:342.
4. Gusberg SB, Runowicz CD. Gynecologic cancers. In: Holleb AI, Fink DJ, Murphy GP, eds. *Clinical Oncology.* Atlanta, Ga: American Cancer Society; 1991:481-497.
5. Young JL Jr, Miller RW. Incidence of malignant tumors in U.S. children. *J Pediatr.* 1975;86:254.
6. Boring CC, Squires TS, Tong T. Cancer statistics 1992. *CA.* 1992;9:42.
7. Schottenfeld D, Fraumeni JF Jr, eds. *Cancer Epidemiology and Prevention.* Philadelphia, Pa: WB Saunders Co; 1982.
8. Henderson BE. Establishment of an association between a virus and a human cancer. *J Natl Cancer Inst.* 1989;81:320.
9. Levine PH, Ablashi DV, Nunuyama M, et al, eds. *Epstein-Barr Virus and Human Disease.* Clifton, NJ: Humana Press; 1987.
10. McNab JCM, Walkinshaw SA, Cordiner JW, Clements JB. Human papillomavirus in clinically and histologically normal tissue of patients with genital cancer. *N Engl J Med.* 1986;315:1052.
11. Bunn PA Jr, Schecter GP, Jaffe E, et al. Clinical course of retrovirus-associated adult T-cell lymphoma in the United States. *N Engl J Med.* 1983;309:256.
12. Buice JD, Fraumeni JF Jr, eds. *Radiation Carcinogenesis: Epidemiology and Biological Significance.* New York, NY: Raven Press; 1984.
13. Urbach F. Geographic distribution of skin cancer. *J Surg Oncol.* 1971; 3:219.
14. Weisburger JH, Horn CL. The causes of cancer. In: Holleb AI, Fink DJ, Murphy GP, eds. *Clinical Oncology.* Atlanta, Ga: American Cancer Society; 1991:80-98.
15. Rosen PP, Braun DW, Kinne DR. The clinical significance of preinvasive breast cancer. *Cancer.* 1980; 46-919.
16. Coleman N. Secondary malignancy after treatment for Hodgkin's disease: an evolving picture. *J Clin Oncol.* 1986;4:821.
17. Cooper MR, Cooper MR. Principles of medical oncology. In: Holleb AI, Fink DJ, Murphy GP, eds. *Clinical Oncology.* Atlanta, Ga: American Cancer Society; 1991:47-68.

COMMON ISSUES FACING ADULTS WITH CANCER

Catherine S. Cordoba, MSW, ACSW
Patricia Fobair, MSW, MPH, LCSW
David B. Callan, MSW

Of all life events, a cancer diagnosis is one of the most startling and disturbing. With this unpleasant surprise, life suddenly changes. Although the person with a new diagnosis may have been feeling perfectly healthy, in an instant the future becomes uncertain. The words of one patient put the experience in perspective: "To me, cancer is a monster–like the bogeyman in the closet. You never expect to see it, and all of a sudden, there it is."[1]

"Why me?" is a poignant question frequently asked by cancer patients. However, "Why not?" is a more rational query, considering that 30% of persons living today eventually will have some type of cancer.[2]

The impact of cancer can be tremendous. The way a person functions, his or her ability to continue working or to perform the same work, marital and family relationships, educational plans, career advancement, financial stability, social relationships, life-style, and value systems can all be disrupted.[3] Cancer challenges self-esteem and a person's sense of pride.

Cancer is a chronic disease with psychosocial consequences. However favorable the outcome, the specter of death presents itself. As the events that follow a diagnosis rapidly unfold, the person may begin to feel that life is out of control. In order to be most helpful to and effective with cancer patients and their families, social workers need to understand what cancer is (and is not) and what treatment consists of as well as the psychosocial issues and the common concerns of persons who experience cancer. Social workers must work from knowledge, not just from intuition or feelings of compassion and empathy. Systematic inquiry into problems and needs from the patient's point of view is necessary so that the real needs can be met.

Cancer involves a complex set of changing conditions that have both a history and a future. Issues in the cancer continuum include:

- The threat to survival and the physical, emotional, and intimacy issues that are involved
- The changes in values and outlook on life and the spiritual and philosophical aspects of the experience
- The social, financial, and physical resources regarding the costs of cancer, employment, discrimination, insurance, and the health care system itself.

By focusing on these areas, social workers can intervene to help cancer patients and their families reduce stress and become more confident in their ability to maintain a sense of control.

ISSUES INVOLVED IN THE THREAT TO SURVIVAL

A major emotional theme of cancer is the uncertainty about outcome. Even though the trusted surgeon may say "We got it all," an individual may be haunted by the fear that a stray cell has wandered off to continue the growth of cancer. Cancer has been compared to the sword of Damocles,[4] ever-present, ready to fall at any time. Life is not certain for anyone, but this is particularly true for someone who has or has had cancer. Because the course of the disease for most patients is unpredictable, a cautionary note is appropriate: Social workers considering working in the field of oncology need to be comfortable with ambiguity since this is what cancer patients and their families must live with.

KEY STRESS PERIODS

Key stress periods in the cancer continuum include:

- The time of diagnosis. This includes the time a person first becomes aware of a symptom or warning sign.
- The treatment period. Treatment usually generates high levels of anxiety.
- The end of treatment and period of remission. This often means a loss of support from health care professionals and the patient's entrance into a period of uncertainty. Issues of survivorship become paramount.

- Recurrence of cancer. At this time an individual becomes fully aware of his or her mortality.
- The terminal phase.

THE TIME OF DIAGNOSIS

The moment can be heart-stopping when a person notices a warning sign such as a lump that could mean she or he has cancer. The discovery may be followed by denial and a delay in seeking treatment, or it may prompt the individual to immediately seek medical attention.

A biopsy, or the removal of tissue or fluid from the body for diagnostic examination, is done to establish whether a cancer is present. This involves waiting for laboratory reports and consequently can be a time of excruciating anxiety for the person awaiting the results.

A cancer diagnosis produces feelings of shock, anger, grief, and uncertainty that can be compounded by inadequate communication with medical personnel. The new patient may be so overwhelmed that he or she does not really hear what is being said.

The doctor-patient relationship is extremely important at this time. It is during the initial encounters when the diagnosis is confirmed that the physician has the opportunity to establish a trusting relationship that is so important to the successful mastery of the cancer experience.

The increasing emphasis on patients' rights and more-informed patients has changed the way diagnosis and treatment unfold. Rather than the physician alone deciding what is to be done when the diagnosis is made, the patient is given the opportunity to take an active role in learning about choices and deciding treatment modalities. This is often clearer in theory than in practice, however, as a great deal of unfamiliar and complicated information has to be assimilated in a short time. These decisions have far-reaching consequences and are often based on limited knowledge. Decisions also are affected by the degree of stress the person is experiencing. When there are multiple treatment options, patients often feel reassured when the physician is able to offer a clear and definitive recommendation.

While time is of the essence in the treatment of cancer, a short interval between a diagnosis confirming cancer and the initiation of treatment to allow the patient to learn more about his or her disease and the available treatment choices usually will not be detrimental to outcome.

THE TREATMENT PERIOD

The patient and family may experience a great deal of stress in trying to cope with complex medical and physical issues in addition to the need to relate to a bewildering array of physicians and other health professionals. During this phase, some patients will develop a sense that they are dealing with a disease process out of their control. Dependency on those providing treatment can result in feelings of a loss of personal control and self-esteem.

Aggressive and intensive treatment regimens, often administered in large medical centers far from the patient's home, pose additional psychosocial challenges. The logistics of getting to and from treatment may consume an enormous amount of time and energy.

Physical Effects

People with cancer can experience a wide variety of physical effects from the disease and from the treatment they undergo. Changes in the body constitute insults to personal integrity, self-concept, and identity.

Yasko and Greene[5] have identified a full range of symptoms or problems due to the cancer itself, to treatment, or to psychological reactions. These include: anemia, bleeding tendency, constipation, diarrhea, difficulty swallowing, dry mouth, itchy skin, fatigue, nausea and vomiting, hair loss, loss of appetite, mouth and throat sores, respiratory problems, sexual and reproductive problems, skin reactions, taste alterations, urinary tract problems, lymphedema (swelling), infection, and pain.

These physical problems can have a serious impact on a patient's quality of life and, in some cases, may cause patients to question the value of treatment. There are antidotes for most of these symptoms and side effects and social workers can support patients in seeking symptomatic relief from the treatment team.

Factors Affecting Patient Adjustment

The treatment modality and the extent of disease may determine the physical outcome for patients.[6] Physical adjustment following the diagnosis generally is linked most closely with side effects of treatment.[7,8] The toxic effects of treatment associated with chemotherapy or radiation therapy are factors influencing physical adaptation. Cassileth and coworkers[9] found that the frequency of actual side effects was much greater than patients originally anticipated. While psychological factors were found to play a role, the nature and severity of side effects were more influenced by physiological factors.

Changes in energy level, activity, body image, and self-concept are also related to treatment side effects. A significant proportion of patients experience energy loss, fatigue, and loss of libido following treatment. Patients with self-reported energy loss were more likely to be depressed.[10] Leisure activities were more affected by the cancer experience than work activities.[11] Patients who were treated with radiation only were less likely to report a change in sexual interest than patients treated with radiation and chemotherapy.[11]

Results of studies with breast cancer patients on the physical effects of surgical procedures support the positive psychosocial effects of "lesser" rather than "greater" surgery. Women who underwent lumpectomies rather than mastectomies reported fewer feelings of lessened attractiveness and femininity, were less self-conscious about their appearance, received more emotional support from friends, and were more open about their surgeries and their sexual feelings after surgery.[12]

Mages et al.[13] identified three important variables in adapting to cancer. They are:

1. Severity of illness
2. Psychological stability
3. Social supports.

These variables were associated with changes in self-image, mood, personal relationships, sexual life, assertiveness, and work.

No psychosocial factor consistently has been associated with length of survival or remission. Rather, surviving cancer appears to be closely linked to inherent biological and physiological processes within the individual and inherent in the disease.[7,9,14]

Sexual Functioning

Sexual functioning is a concern for many persons with cancer, which can affect sexuality in the following ways:[15]

- By the disease process, either through damage directly to primary sexual organs or their nerve supplies or through weakness and debilitation

- By treatment, which can result in temporary or permanent sexual alteration or dysfunction
- By body image alterations or cosmetic side effects following surgery or other treatment
- By anxiety, depression, and other psychologic disorders
- By reactions of significant others.

Body-altering surgeries resulting in loss or impairment of vital organs can have a powerful effect on sexual functioning. Many surgical procedures have an impact on body image and self-esteem. Any insult to body image creates a high-risk situation for sexual dysfunction.[16]

Chemotherapy can produce impotence or sterility in men, premature menopausal symptoms in women, and decreased libido in both sexes. Treatment-related nausea can be a deterrent to sexual interest. Some head and neck operations may eliminate the ability to kiss or engage in other oral activity.[16]

Cancer and its consequences can be sexually inhibiting. Feelings about having cancer affect ways a cancer patient may relate to a sexual partner. The patient may feel he or she will be exposed as incomplete, damaged, or dying; these feelings may lead to inhibition or abstention from sexual activity.[16] Shame and embarrassment can affect intimacy. Sexual partners may be fearful of hurting the patient or may be "turned off" by a partner's abdominal stoma or stomal breathing during intercourse.[16]

In studies comparing women with cancer to women without cancer, women with cancer reported experiencing significant sexual dysfunction and reported becoming sexually inactive. The degree of sexual functioning often correlates with the magnitude of the treatment.[17]

Sexual problems of women who have had mastectomies for breast cancer have been reported extensively. Common concerns are a sense of having been mutilated, loss of feelings of femininity, and fear of death. A woman experiencing these feelings will usually see herself as less acceptable as a sexual partner. The sexuality of the male partner after a woman's mastectomy may be affected as well and may result in a decrease in the frequency of activity.[16]

Patients with testicular cancer also experience sexual difficulties. Men with sexual impairment reported more psychological symptoms, strained intimate relations, and negative changes in other areas of life functioning after treatment for nonseminomatous testicular cancer.[18]

Testicular cancer patients, compared to men without the disease, reported less sexual activity, lower sexual desire, more erectile dysfunction, more difficulty achieving orgasm, reduced orgasmic intensity, and reduced semen volume. Sterility was a frequent source of anxiety for one-quarter of the men.[19]

Significant sexual deterioration was seen in three groups of men treated for prostate cancer with radiotherapy, orchiectomy, and estrogen. Men subjected to orchiectomy or estrogen treatment were seldom capable of having intercourse or of experiencing orgasm, while more than one-half of the men receiving radiation had marked reduction in frequency of sexual activity. Men treated with estrogen had higher depression scores than those in the other two treatment groups, possibly due to the associated changes in body image produced.[20]

Summary of Treatment Effects

Social workers will find that cancer patients' physical problems range from minimal loss of energy and fatigue to poorly managed pain and terminal illness. In large degree, physical problems reflect the nature and duration of treatment as well as an individual's inherent physiology. Although reactions to treatment are individual and unpredictable, in general, the more intense the treatment, the greater the patient's difficulty. Good oncologic care requires as much attention to the management of side effects as the control of the disease.

THE END OF TREATMENT, REMISSION, AND SURVIVORSHIP

Cancer patients may mark off the days until their treatment comes to an end, but the cessation of treatment may bring about an unsettling period. Patients may have functioned so long in a protected environment, in constant contact with health professionals who monitored their progress and provided support, that they may feel anxious and uncertain at the completion of therapy. Relatively minor aches and pains may cause them to feel the cancer has returned; concern about health becomes paramount. Although much of this dissipates with time, the "Damocles syndrome"[4] lingers.

The extent of disease and/or treatment has a major impact on the patient's energy, activity, body image, or sexual activity during or following treatment. For example, recovery from a lumpectomy should be less complicated than recovery from a colon resection. Sometimes physical recovery does not progress as smoothly as one might expect. The social worker's skill in understanding the patient's psychosocial adaptation is vital to the patient as well as to the team in its ability to maximize the fullest recovery possible.

With the culmination of successful treatment against cancer, the person leaves the role of "patient" for that of "survivor." Much may be different now–bodily functions, sexual and intimate relationships, values, outlook on life, and (perhaps) economic well-being. The ability to work as before or to resume former activities may be altered. Problems with employment and insurance, discussed later, may become of paramount importance. Some may feel they always will have the burden of being an ex-cancer patient. Life has changed, indeed.

There is increasing recognition of survivorship needs, and a number of groups or organizations focus on them. The National Coalition for Cancer Survivorship is one. A newsletter called "Surviving" is published by the Department of Radiation Oncology at Stanford University Hospital. Many units of the American Cancer Society participate in special events for survivors. As more people survive cancer, even more attention will be given to the issues raised in its aftermath.

RECURRENCE AND TERMINAL ILLNESS

For many patients, the knowledge that cancer has recurred can be devastating. Many patients see recurrence as the beginning of the end. While this is not necessarily so, recurrence often means more aggressive treatment. In addition to the physical phenomena, patients must deal with the overwhelming assault on their hope for cure. For many patients, recurrence signifies the first real challenge to survival. This has been described by many patients as a more serious crisis than the initial diagnosis. While most patients, with adequate support, are able to deal with this there are some who will respond with a desperate search for unorthodox treatments.

With advancing disease, many patients fear abandonment, being alone, or suffering intractable pain. The support of family, friends, and health professionals becomes increasingly important. The patient needs to know that he or she will not be abandoned by loved ones and that health professionals can be counted on for assistance in functioning at an optimal level without pain.

Pain

Persistent pain is one of the most feared physical responses to cancer, although pain does not seem to be a significant problem for the majority of patients in the early stages of the disease. When metastatic disease is present, however, about one-third of the patients report significant pain.[21]

Advances in pain management have now resulted in the ability to control most cancer pain. However, this new technology is not being universally applied. The advocacy skills of social workers can be well utilized in helping patients access specialists in pain management.

The psychosocial assessment skills of the social worker are crucial to the health care team's understanding of this complex area. For example, patients and families often bring inaccurate information about addiction, tolerance, and treatment side effects that seriously compromise effective pain control.

The social worker with good supportive counseling skills can take advantage of opportunities to learn basic behavioral management techniques that are often quite helpful to this group of patients.

Quality of Life and Advanced Disease

During this period the quality-of-life concept becomes crucial. The patient, no matter how ill, still has a life to lead and it should be one that still holds joy and happiness.

Some patients whose cancer has recurred speak of themselves as terminal cancer patients. While some of the uncertainty about their cancer is gone, with treatment they may live for many more years. These patients should be referred to as having advanced cancer rather than terminal cancer and they should be encouraged to live their lives as fully as possible. Most people have unfinished business in their lives and persons with advanced disease should settle it if they are able. Doing so can bring a patient much satisfaction and help in maintaining some feelings of control.

A great deal has been said about patients going through the "stages" of dying. However, stages are fluid and each patient faces death in his or her own way. Individuals can be helped to face death with courage and dignity, but the decisions are theirs to make. Some individuals may see death as a welcome relief from the burden of illness and a peaceful transition; others may never give up fighting, choosing to battle cancer to the end.

Emotional Factors

The major fears that accompany cancer have been characterized as the "five D's"–death, disability, disfigurement, dependence, and disruption of key relationships. The fears, which are normal, center first around the threat to life and then the threat to the quality of life.[22]

As with most chronic illnesses, cancer is a family disease in the sense that the whole family is affected by it in some way. One often-overlooked aspect of cancer is the significant number of families in which more than one member has or has had cancer. Two members may be receiving treatment at the same time, there may have been a recent death due to cancer, or there may be an unusual number of cancers in the same family. Because these families are under considerable stress and face additional emotional burdens, social workers should query about any other illnesses, particularly cancer, in the family.[1]

Once an individual has moved beyond the initial crisis of diagnosis, a variety of cognitive, behavioral, and emotional patterns begin to emerge. How the person responds emotionally to the sense of personal loss of good health is central to the overall experience. Anxiety, anger, depression, isolation, and guilt are common emotional reactions.

Emotional Adjustment to the Cancer Experience

Several researchers have found that the most important unmet need of cancer patients was for help in dealing with emotional problems.[23,24] Studies indicated that many patients were unaware of resources such as social work assistance within treatment centers and consequently did not indicate a need for help. Therefore, social workers need to find ways of identifying patients and families who might benefit from their intervention.

Because "Why me?" is such a frequent concern to those with cancer, the social worker should explore with them this unsettling question fairly early on. Looking at answers in initial contacts enables patients to have some control of this previously unconscious or preconscious material and, therefore, tends to help them feel less victimized.

Patients' distress and emotional reactions following cancer diagnoses have steered clinical research toward efforts to understand the normal emotional and mood adjustment patterns.

In recent studies, cancer patients' depression scores did not differ significantly from other populations with which they were compared.

Greater depression scores could be accounted for by a number of factors including a recent diagnosis; loss of energy; a younger age; sicker, more disabled patients; and more advanced disease.[10,25-27] Depression scores returned to normal for most patients following treatment, and as a group cancer patients seen in follow-up resembled the normal population in mood.[10,28]

In order to appreciate a patient's emotional response, it is necessary to have a basic understanding of the nature of depression. Some patients are misdiagnosed as depressed when they are experiencing a normal reaction to a life crisis. Others are assumed to be depressed as a natural consequence of their cancer diagnosis. There will be some patients who bring a pre-existing clinical depression to the cancer experience. Others may develop serious symptomatology as a result of severe physical and emotional distress.

Social workers need to be knowledgeable about the normal emotional response to crisis and the clinical symptoms of a major depressive disorder requiring psychiatric consultation and/or medication. All members of the health care team must be aware of those situations in which depression results from an organic rather than psychological phenomenon.

FACTORS INFLUENCING INDIVIDUAL AND FAMILY RESPONSES TO CANCER

The social worker's understanding of the common issues affecting cancer patients and their families needs to be supplemented with knowledge of factors that influence responses to a cancer crisis. Age, socioeconomic status, coping styles, family functioning, and cultural or religious identity are among the psychosocial factors that contribute to the meaning of cancer to the individual and to subsequent adaptation.

AGE

An individual's age at the time of a cancer diagnosis can be a significant determinant of coping responses. Childhood cancer can pose major interruptions in a child's developmental stages, his or her relationships with peers, and progress in school. The adolescent's drive toward independence and mastery may be halted by the need for increased dependence on parents and health care professionals. At a time when individuation and separation from parents are appropriate, the teenager may be pulled in the opposite direction. Children and teenagers must be helped to live as normally as possible and to stay in school as much as possible. Future risks to health and well being as a result of treatment have to be considered.

Young adults face a different set of challenges in a cancer crisis. Their main life-cycle tasks–establishing themselves in the world of work, forming intimate relationships, setting up a household, raising a family–can be seriously obstructed by an occurrence of cancer. Ability to work or to advance in a career may be seriously impaired. Parents may be asked to resume roles as caretakers that can destabilize a young household and freshly formed relationships. For example, parents may assume that they, rather than the patient's spouse, are the primary relatives when it comes to consulting with physicians.

Older adults may find it necessary to become dependent in varying degrees and may find it difficult to carry out their responsibilities. Their livelihood and intimate relationships may be affected. The occurrence of cancer at retirement age can frustrate expectations of pleasurable activities, and the financial burden may seriously jeopardize retirement savings. Recent retirees can feel cheated when cancer interferes with their carefully prepared retirement plans.

The prevalence of cancer increases in the elderly. This oldest group may have special circumstances that exacerbate their situation when a major illness occurs. There may be no spouse, family member, or friend able to provide support and care. Anxiety over the cost of care may be acute, and the person may be coping also with other chronic illnesses and debilitation. However, the occurrence of cancer can accelerate the natural process of life review, the accomplishment of unfinished business, and the process of self-acceptance.

SOCIOECONOMIC STATUS

Cancer, as will be delineated later in this chapter, is a very costly illness in many ways; and its burdens fall more heavily on those at the lower end of the socioeconomic scale. Many of the "working poor" lack employment-related benefits such as pay for sick leave and health insurance. The crisis of cancer is compounded by the simultaneous threat to other survival needs such as food and housing. Middle-class families can become impoverished and see their hopes for advanced education for their children and a comfortable old age disappear. Adults who have been self-supporting all their lives may have to undergo the trauma of applying for some type of public assistance.

Affluent families can be relatively free of financial worries and able to ameliorate some of the secondary effects of the illness by obtaining adequate assistance in their homes, counseling services, special clothing or equipment, and anxiety-reducing appliances such as intercom systems.

Families in rural areas often encounter special hardships entering complex health care systems that may be quite distant from their homes. They may feel forced into an unfamiliar medical system characterized by organized hierarchies of professionals, sophisticated and impersonal technologies, medical jargon, and confusing means of payment. All this can heighten anxiety when the patient and family may feel they have already lost control of their lives because of cancer.

COPING STYLES

The influence of personality on coping style is very complex. Some individuals prefer to deal with a crisis by turning first within themselves to clarify their thoughts and feelings; only later can these thoughts and feelings be shared with others. Others respond by first seeking conversation with others; for them the process of sharing thoughts and feelings is a means of achieving clarity.

Some patients prefer to gather exhaustive information about their cancer and its treatment as they progress through the continuum. Because seeking and obtaining information helps them to attain feelings of control and mastery over their situation, they will read as much as they can and question the medical team continuously. Others find that a lot of information increases their anxiety; they prefer not to question but to place all their trust in the medical team. The challenge for the treatment team is to strike a balance between the information that must be given as part of informed consent and the patient's comfort level.

People differ in their ability to accept support from others. Some are able to draw strength from other cancer patients like themselves, some rely on their family, and others seek support from health professionals in the medical center. People vary in their ability to tolerate and manage uncertainty. Patients whose natural approach to life's problems is through organization and control seem to adapt less easily to the inherent uncertainties of cancer than do those more congenial to the unexpected elements of life.

There is a wide range of coping styles and it is important to identify adaptive and effective or maladaptive and ineffective coping responses as early as possible. A cancer diagnosis usually seems to be more easily managed by those with a pre-existing ability to adapt to life's challenges than by those who already have dysfunctional coping habits, but there are exceptions.

FAMILY FUNCTIONING STYLE

Cancer impacts not just the patient but the whole family; a cancer diagnosis can upset the equilibrium of an entire household. Therefore, psychosocial cancer care often encompasses the family, not just the patient.

The first impulse for some families facing a cancer diagnosis is to protect each other, and particularly the patient, by maintaining silence. In a misguided effort to shelter the patient (who is most likely very aware of her or his condition) by avoiding a discussion of feelings and problems, the family may isolate the patient who then can become very lonely. The longer such silence continues, the more likely there will be serious difficulty as family members find themselves cut off from one another at a time when they most need each other's support. The social worker needs to facilitate family communication by verbalizing some of the common feelings experienced by patients and families and encouraging families to develop ways to communicate with one another about their feelings and about ways to handle problems.

Sometimes families focus so much attention on the person with cancer that the well members are emotionally and socially neglected. Children are enormously sensitive to changes in the availability of their parents as primary caregivers and may act out their feelings in problem behavior at school and in the home. They may get into fights, neglect schoolwork, have nightmares, develop somatic complaints such as stomachaches or headaches, or regress. Teenagers may engage in risk-taking behavior such as reckless driving or running away from home. Participation in peer support activities, particularly recreation, and individual or family counseling can help well children in a family facing cancer by diminishing the need for acting-out behavior.

Some families operate as "closed" systems by which they rely mostly on their own resources to maintain equilibrium. Others may operate as "open" systems and readily turn to outside resources to maintain their balance. The private style of functioning tends to devalue outside help and these families may resist any form of community support. "Open" families may be better able to cope with cancer since few family units in today's society have sufficient means to cope with a major illness such as cancer totally on their own.

Each family has its own rules and roles that govern the interactions among its members as it attempts to find a new equilibrium in a crisis. Flexibility about these unwritten rules and roles generally fosters adaptive coping. When options are closed about who does what, dysfunctional coping patterns often result. Rigidity about roles and rules are often at the base of a family's maladaptive coping responses.

Every family's coping style is influenced by its prior history of handling stress, especially if the new situation resembles the old one. The legacy of family functioning in past crises is a powerful influence on roles and behaviors. If responses in prior history were adaptive and if the current predicament resembles the earlier one, the coping skills learned at that time will be an asset. However, if the current situation is unlike the earlier one or if coping was maladaptive, the prior history of coping may be a liability to family functioning.

In summary, families who seem to function at an optimum level during a cancer crises know how to communicate painful facts and feelings among themselves, are open to outside support, and are flexible about adapting family roles and rules.

CULTURAL AND RELIGIOUS IDENTITY

The influence of ethnic or religious identity is closely connected with the family's functioning style. Cultural and religious backgrounds help give shape to the meaning that events such as major illness hold for people. They provide a context within which individuals and families interpret what befalls them.

In some cultures, cancer is regarded as a source of shame and its presence in certain parts of the body may be assigned specialized meanings of shame. This view reinforces maladaptive patterns of denial or refusal to share feelings about the disease and often leads to delay in seeking medical help until the cancer is far advanced. Negative interpretations about cancer are not limited to underdeveloped cultures. Contemporary American culture tends to blame the victim for falling prey to cancer.

Religious traditions contribute their own interpretations to a catastrophic illness such as cancer: as a curse, a blessing, a test of virtue, or a warning to change one's ways. An individual's belief about a cancer occurrence may be formulated within the context of these religious traditions.

Because religion by its nature exists in groups and not merely in individuals, it also helps to shape group responses to illness. By and large, religious traditions encourage a compassionate response to illness. A subgroup within a church or synagogue may make a ministry of helping patients and their families. Some religious bodies may sponsor hospitals or hospices in the community. These actions, in turn, form a specialized environment in which patients and the community itself come to interpret the experience of illness.

PERSONAL AND SOCIAL VALUES OF CANCER PATIENTS AND SOCIETY

A patient's assessment of his or her world following a cancer diagnosis is affected by his or her value system and by the view's of the larger society. The value of one's life as a healthy individual must shift to incorporate life altered by cancer.

ARE CANCER PATIENTS "DIFFERENT"?

Although individuals with cancer often are viewed as "different" from others, cancer patients tend to be emotionally healthy individuals whose adjustment problems result primarily from their physical illness.[4] Any differences arise from how persons with cancer view themselves and how others view them.

In spite of greater knowledge about the disease, greater openness, and greater public access to information, myths and misconceptions about cancer still abound. The disease engenders much fear and still carries a stigma.

STIGMA

Because of the stigma associated with cancer, the illness can create feelings of shame and a need for secrecy. Many cancer patients question whether they brought the disease upon themselves because of personality traits, attitudes, past indiscretions, or dissolute life-style.

Stahly[29] interviewed cancer patients to assess the psychosocial adaptation involved in coping with the experience of stigma. Her work was based on the idea that most people believe the world is rational and fair and that people generally get what they deserve. That is, in the long run, good things happen to good people and bad things happen to bad people. Consequently, when something bad happens, the victim's character or behavior is blamed.

There are fairly pervasive feelings, usually below the level of awareness, that the one with cancer must have been guilty of sinful behavior to be punished with a terrible disease like cancer. Social workers should be prepared to explore these irrational ideas with patients.

PERSONALITY FACTORS AND STRESS

The view that the brain controls the body's susceptibility to illness and that an emotional state can alter the body's hormonal and immune system may cause patients to wonder if their emotions played a part in initiating or promoting their cancer. Research to date does not support this. However, the view that emotional distress can lower immunity to some diseases is very different from the view that emotions cause disease.

A prevalent belief–that personality factors and stress play major roles in the etiology of cancer–is often reinforced in the popular press and by some mental health professionals. However, theories about cancer-prone personalities are without scientific basis. Several studies examining emotional issues refute the role of emotion as a powerful initiator in cancer. Neither early signs of depression nor stress were found to be associated with cancer incidence or mortality in three databases from large populations.[30-32]

Simple relationships between psychological states or traits and cancer outcomes have not been identified. Most psychosocial researchers hold that the disease itself is responsible for behavior, not that personality causes the disease. Clearly, more and better research in this area is indicated.

CHANGING PERCEPTIONS AFTER CANCER

Following diagnosis and treatment, many patients report a greater appreciation of time, life, and relationships. Patients describe conscious reordering of priorities to focus on essentials rather than the mundane.

In a personal reflection on his own cancer experience, Mullan[33] (a physician) described that during his treatment period, his view of himself was challenged by the quality of his life, which had been severely compromised. The ever-present possibility of death forced him into a physical and mental struggle with the cancer, the treatment, and the large-scale disruption in his life. In Mullan's cancer experience, survival became not one condition but many.

Following treatment, Mullan said that he wondered when he could safely declare victory over his disease. "There was no moment of cure but rather an evolution from the phase of extended survival into a period when the activity of the disease or the likelihood of its return is sufficiently small that cancer can now be considered permanently arrested,"[33] he wrote. Mullan came to value challenge in finding ways of mapping the middle ground of survivorship and minimizing the medical and social hazards for cancer patients.

In a study of attitudes and value changes of 403 people who had been treated for Hodgkin's disease, Fobair et al.[10] found a number of self-reported value changes. One-hundred-seventy-six patients responded with answers indicating a change in their philosophical meaning in life; 92 viewed changes in their self-concept as the most important factor; and 89 patients felt they had experienced many changes in their view of the importance of relationships. These responses, summarized from unpublished data, are presented in Table 1.

HOPE

Hope is a crucial component for successful adaptation to cancer. The level of hope and ability in coping are interconnected. Hope is influenced by one's religious beliefs, family values, personal goals, and sense of well being. Regardless of prognosis, it is the health care team's responsibility to help the patient preserve realistic hope. What starts out as hope for cure may change over time to hope for more short-term goals.

Pervasive hopelessness is one of the risk factors for suicide. If social work intervention in support of the mobilization of the patient's hope is unsuccessful, then psychiatric consultation should be considered.

SOCIAL SUPPORTS

Considerable evidence exists that a positive adjustment to a cancer diagnosis, treatment, and survival is affected by social, marital, and professional support. Bloom's study of social support as a predictor of adjustment to breast cancer pointed out that patients' perceptions of

Table 1
ATTITUDES AND VALUE CHANGES REPORTED BY HODGKIN'S DISEASE PATIENTS †

Philosophical Changes
"I have a greater understanding of the meaning of life."
"I appreciate life more."
"My values have deepened."
"I have reviewed my life in greater detail."
"I have more religious feelings about the meaning of life."
Self-Concept Changes
"I feel stronger and more self-confident."
"I feel more mature."
"I now recognize my personal mortality."
"I am more aware of my human frailty."
"I have resolved my problems with ambitions versus energy."
"I have a sense of having grown up earlier."
"My sense of personal concept is stronger."
Relationship Changes
"I now experience closer relationships with my family."
"I know who loves me."
"I am more willing to accept others as they are."
"I believe in taking care of others more now."
"I appreciated the professional and medical care I received."

† Respondents were asked the question, "What benefits, if any, have there been to having gone through the experience of Hodgkin's disease?"

family cohesiveness and amount of social contact directly affected how well they coped and felt adjusted.[34]

A study of breast cancer patients indicated that women who adjusted the best also had the highest levels of family cohesion.[35] Northouse[36] found that patients and husbands who reported higher levels of social support also experienced fewer adjustment difficulties.

Cancer patients often express feelings of being alone with their illness and of social isolation. Contributing to stress is the cancer stigma, which is a significant manifestation of the isolation and the withdrawal of social support. Stahly[29] found that young patients were more likely than older patients to spontaneously mention embarrassment and shame about their illness. Social stress also appeared to be further heightened for patients whose prognosis was poor; terminal-stage patients were among those scoring highest on a stigma inventory.[29]

Stahly also found aspects of social stress that added to the stigmatization of the cancer patient. For example, when the patient is seen as helpless and the disease as powerful and out of control, others may respond to the patient with discomfort and social distance.[33] Patients often must bear the burden of being referred to as "cancer victims." This label diminishes them since they are viewed as passive recipients of whatever life hands them.

Some prevalent notions in our society are that persons are the masters of their fate, that they can control what happens by sheer force of will, and that any obstacle can be overcome. In this sense, society holds its members culpable for their diseases, especially when the disease is cancer. The social environment, rather than being supportive, can be oppressive to persons with cancer.

In general, cancer patients are normal people under a great deal of stress, some of which can emanate from their social networks. These patients are vulnerable to the stress produced not only by negative attitudes of significant people in their lives, but also by their own negative attitudes. It is especially important that social workers monitor their own attitudes so that they do not unwittingly add to the patient's sense of isolation.

The ability to reframe cancer into a more positive experience rather than a solely negative one stems from one of the most sophisticated coping strategies available.[37] Patients who are able to successfully implement this reframing report spiritual enrichment, increased appreciation of each day, and greater intimacy with loved ones.

There seems to be a basic spiritual need to find meaning and purpose in life. As a patient's physical condition deteriorates, spiritual issues commonly become more important determinants of quality of life. The prospect of death can bring about a sense of immediacy to living and can lead an individual to regroup personal resources, abilities, and priorities.

Most patients will experience this type of adaptation at various times during their illness. However, it is not necessarily a constant theme and, for some patients, is unachievable at any time.

FINANCES, EMPLOYMENT, AND INSURANCE

Persons with a cancer health history can experience significant problems with finances, insurance, employment, and employment discrimination.

FINANCIAL CONCERNS RELATED TO CANCER

Cancer is a very costly disease. Its costs include the direct expense of diagnosis and treatment and indirect costs related to loss of earnings, earning power, and productivity. The costs to society are enormous and the costs to patients and their families can be catastrophic.

Direct Costs

As many as 37 million people in the United States are not covered by any form of health insurance. This group includes people employed by small businesses, the self-employed, part-time workers, persons who have opted for early retirement, persons whose circumstances have changed due to divorce, and others. A significant number of poor people are not covered by the Medicaid program. These uninsured people stand to lose everything in the event of an illness such as cancer. In other instances, costly premiums have forced some low-income families to choose between subsistence and insurance. It is ironic that those with the least resources have the poorest coverage.[27]

Millions more Americans have inadequate coverage. They may have insurance that will cover much of the cost of hospitalization but none for outpatient care. Cancer is being treated increasingly on an outpatient basis, so the costs of treatment and follow-up care can place an enormous burden on many patients and families. A major illness can deplete savings and place the family's financial survival in jeopardy. Some families have to mortgage the future of their children to pay for health care; in this sense, cancer can be catastrophic in more ways than one.

While the patient is absorbed in concerns about illness and treatment, family members may be struggling with financial worries. Feelings of guilt about concerns over expenses are common.

Indirect Costs

Indirect costs include the costs of getting to and from treatment which can be significant. Major treatment centers often are located far from patients' homes, necessitating long drives and perhaps lodging expenses.

Gasoline, meals away from home, housing, car repair and maintenance expenses, and charges for baby-sitters are other indirect costs. Patients also may require special equipment and clothing, prostheses, and wigs; nursing care; assistance with activities of daily living, child care, or household chores; special meals or diet supplements; and other assistance. The promise of new treatment methods or a new research protocol may prompt families to risk all their resources in the hope of saving the patient's life. The whole family may be uprooted in order to go to another part of the country, leaving jobs and familiar support networks behind. Families may arrive on the doorstep of the treatment center with no money and no place to stay, but with the faith that they can work things out for the patient's benefit. Social workers can assist the family in adequate planning that can prevent such situations from happening.

Resource Interventions

Many patients are unaware they may be eligible for certain public programs and often know little of other community resources. Social workers in oncology need to be knowledgeable about resources in order to be most helpful to over-extended families. Although finances can be a tremendous source of stress, most people find it difficult to ask for help. Applying for welfare or other kinds of assistance can be a tremendous blow to self-esteem, but social workers can help with this process and with the feelings that accompany it.

Indirect Costs Related to Work and Family

A person with cancer may be unable to work for long periods of time or may lose a job. The patient may be unable physically to resume a former job and may have to seek a different kind of employment. A patient's caretaker may have to take a great deal of time off from work to transport a patient to and from treatment or to provide care. Often, the mother of a child with cancer has to give up a job she needs to support the family in order to care for the ill child.

Cancer places other burdens on the family. Adolescents may have to enter the workforce to contribute to family support. College plans may have to be deferred or given up when a family member has cancer. Recreation or pleasure of any kind is often missing from families dealing with cancer. At a time when well children may need attention and nurturing, their parents may be consumed by the struggles with cancer.

EMPLOYMENT ISSUES

In our society, "the job" is at the center of adult life; an individual's self-image and community status tend to be shaped by how he or she earns a living.[38]

Due to increased survival, employment has become a more pressing cancer issue. Historically, attention was focused on clinical issues and it was assumed that a person with cancer never worked again. The current understanding is that a person with cancer should continue working during treatment, if possible, or should return to work as soon as possible after treatment. Barofsky[39] found that cancer patients who continued working during treatment were more likely to continue working following treatment than those who ceased working. However, the person who has or has had cancer may have difficulty returning to work, particularly in starting a new job.

Who Returns to Work?

"Who returns to work?" and "Who has the most difficulty doing so?" are questions considered by researchers. The stage of the cancer, the aggressiveness of treatment, and the type of work are major prognostic factors influencing the resumption of employment. Patients with limited disease or light occupations more often returned to work than patients with extensive disease or heavy occupations.[40] Other important predictors include coworker support and absence of depression.[41] Disease sites and functional loss also contribute to patients' ability to return to work.[42]

Economic Vulnerability

Groups of people with cancer health histories at greatest risk for work problems are also vulnerable to economic and job climate changes. These groups include:[41]

- Young people with no work history
- Persons with low self-esteem or prior emotional problems
- Persons with notable physical disabilities or treatment side effects
- Patients with advanced disease
- Blue-collar workers
- Low-income, seasonally, and marginally employed persons
- Nonwhites

- Persons age 50 and older
- Persons initiating work transitions.

On the other hand, persons with a positive self-image and coworker support experienced higher return-to-work rates and fewer problems after they returned to work.[10,43]

Employment Discrimination

Job discrimination involves any adverse action taken by any employer in whole or in part because of a person's legally protected status.[44] The instance of discrimination most commonly reported is denial of new job opportunities because of a cancer history. Dismissal from current employment because of cancer, failure to receive earned promotions, curtailment of key work functions or demotion, reductions in employee benefits, and refusal to allow changes in schedules or tasks to accommodate such needs as radiation therapy or chemotherapy have also been reported.[44]

The number of people with cancer health histories who have experienced employment discrimination has been investigated by researchers. Crothers[43] summarized six studies examining patients' job-related discrimination or work-related problems. Percentages of patients in each study reporting job discrimination varied from 13% to 45%.

Discrimination is often subtle. Applicants with a cancer health history may be told a better-qualified candidate has been chosen or be given another seemingly plausible explanation. Aware that a cancer history may hinder a job search, former patients are sometimes faced with a dilemma of whether to tell the truth and risk not being hired or to conceal the truth and hope that it never comes out. Since a pre-employment physical exam often is required, many patients volunteer their cancer histories following a firm job offer.

Personal factors also enter into work-related problems. Some studies of cancer-related work problems found that persons with cancer health histories who show low self-esteem, higher scores of depression, and prior health history of emotional problems are more likely to experience work problems.[10,45]

LEGISLATION

The laws that protect men and women who have had cancer from employment discrimination are most often contained in state and federal provisions protecting the physically handicapped. The major piece of federal legislation in this area is the Vocational Rehabilitation Act of 1973, Sections 503 and 504. The Americans With Disabilities Act gives disabled persons the same civil-rights protection in jobs, accommodations, and services that apply to minorities, women, and the elderly. Employers may not reject applicants or fire current employees on the basis of disability.

A review of state disability laws reveals that individuals with cancer health histories are generally protected from employment discrimination. Many states pattern their definitions of "physical handicap" after the federal provisions of the Vocational Rehabilitation Act of 1973. Several states are considering expanding their discrimination laws to protect people with cancer health histories because the needs of individuals faced with cancer-based discrimination are often not addressed in existing legislation. The accommodation needs of workers with cancer histories may include modified work hours to allow for treatment or follow-up. New statutes should prohibit an employer from requiring an employee to meet standards that surpass or are unrelated to the physical demands of the job.[46]

Assistance With Employment Problems and Rights

Many patients feel their physicians have no awareness of problems they may be having with their work; consequently, they do not bring up the problems unless asked directly. The social worker must be sure these problems are addressed and that persons have the opportunity to discuss their concerns. Work and work-related problems should be discussed during any psychosocial assessment. Patients should be encouraged to remain on the job as much as they are able.

People with cancer health histories need to be informed of their rights. The American Cancer Society can provide information on laws protecting individuals with cancer health histories and material that outlines employment rights and the appeals process. The National Cancer Institute and the National Coalition for Cancer Survivorship also have produced patient education materials that address this subject. (See Suggested Readings section of this chapter.)

In addition to discussing work concerns and informing patients of their rights, social workers can assist patients by providing support groups that offer a forum for sharing and exchanging concerns and experiences.

INSURANCE ISSUES

Obtaining life and health insurance is important to long-term surviving cancer patients, but this can present serious problems. In the Greenleigh Associates study of 810 cancer patients, adequate insurance coverage was a key factor in the financial impact of cancer. Patients with the lowest incomes had the greatest cost burden in obtaining insurance.[23] In a study of 100 adults treated for childhood diseases between 1945 and 1975, Holmes[47] found that cancer survivors had significantly more difficulty than their sibling controls in securing life and health insurance.

Health Insurance

"Health insurance has been transformed from a product for the financially prudent into a vital protection against individual financial catastrophe," according to Marshall-Cohen.[48] The most vulnerable group is labeled as high risk and, therefore, considered uninsurable by the health insurance industry: persons with cancer, heart disease, arthritis, diabetes, and other chronic diseases. Without insurance, these persons are left with the choice of bankruptcy in the event of catastrophic illness or "spending down" to the poverty level in order to be eligible for state Medicaid benefits.

The major barriers to affordable health insurance for people with cancer health histories are:[43]

- Refusal of new applications
- Policy cancellations or reductions
- Higher premiums (especially when converting from group to individual policies)
- Waived or excluded pre-existing disorders
- Extended waiting periods.

In 1982, Burton and Zones estimated that nearly 30% of all Californians with cancer histories who were able to work would encounter insurance problems at some point in their lifetimes.[49] With the dramatic rise in health care costs, this estimate would be higher today.

Mor reported on the problems with insurance coverage that patients experienced at the time of their therapy for cancer. Among 149 patients, 11.5% reported a change in health insurance coverage; 4.5%, cancelled insurance; 2.8%, insurance at its maximum limit; and 20%, insurance covered less than 75% of their medical expenses.[50]

Persons at Greatest Risk

Access to group insurance is much less costly than securing it as an individual; individual health coverage is also difficult to obtain. "Health insurance is considered to be a benefit or compensation connected with a job," according to Crothers.[43] While employment opens the door to health insurance, a number of people are at risk due to minimal or no insurance. These include:[44]

- Low-income families earning $10 000 or less per year
- Nonwhites
- The unemployed
- Involuntary part-time workers
- Seasonally or marginally employed workers
- Blue-collar workers
- Workers in organizations employing 10 or fewer people
- Persons over 65 vulnerable to gaps in Medicare
- Individuals with adverse health histories.

Insurance Options for People With Cancer Histories

Insurance options are described in the American Cancer Society pamphlet, "Cancer: Your Job, Insurance, and the Law," and by Crothers.[44] These options include the following:

1. Obtaining employment with a large company is the surest way to gain access to group insurance. The best type of plan is a so-called guaranteed issue insurance, which provides benefits to all employees regardless of previous health histories.
2. A person who has had hours reduced, quit a job, or been fired since July 1986 and who has worked for an organization employing 20 or more persons should explore insurance conversion privileges mandated through COBRA. This applies to surviving,

divorced, or separated spouses, and dependent children.

3. Persons who are currently employed should not leave their jobs until they have explored conversion options to individual plans from their group plans. However, premiums may be considerably higher and less comprehensive with individual plans, which usually must be applied for within 30 days of termination of employment. Typically, these plans terminate after one year if cancer history is involved.
4. In some areas of the country, Blue Cross/Blue Shield and some health maintenance organizations (HMOs) offer open enrollment periods for individuals during which applications are accepted regardless of prior health history.
5. Group insurance may be available through fraternal, professional, or trade organizations such as those for retired persons, teachers, social workers, and realtors. A guaranteed issue plan should be sought. Parents of school-aged children should explore life insurance available through schools.
6. Persons who have any past military affiliation should inquire about Veterans Administration or CHAMPUS benefits.
7. Eligibility for Medicare should be explored. It covers most people who are 65 or older and persons who are permanently disabled who have been receiving Social Security benefits for approximately two years.
8. Persons in low-income brackets or who are unemployed may be eligible for local or state benefits such as Medicaid. Some patients with very limited assets and very high medical expenses also may be eligible for Medicaid benefits after a certain level of expenses is reached.
9. An independent insurance broker may be able to locate a benefit package. Group insurance is preferable to individual insurance.

A few states have initiated catastrophic health insurance programs. Premiums can be big, but usually cannot exceed a mandated ceiling (an average of 200% of applicable standard rates). Twenty-three states maintain high-risk pools for people unaccepted by insurance carriers; the rules vary from state to state. A few other states have established an all-payor rate-setting system that includes an allowance for bad debts and charity. Limited expansion of Medicaid eligibility in the form of federal grants to meet uncompensated health care costs allows greater participation of currently excluded groups.[43]

Insurance and Treatment Choices

Aspects of a patient's insurance that involve additional costs can affect access to medical care. Several studies have highlighted the importance of insurance in determining patients' and physicians' choice of and initiation of treatment.

In a comparison of cancer diagnoses and commencement of treatment, Greenwold found that patients who made copayments waited an average of 1.25 months longer between initial suspicion of illness and obtaining a definitive diagnosis than those with full insurance coverage. Time after diagnosis until the beginning of treatment averaged 0.83 months longer for HMO members than for those in fee-for-service insurance plans.[51]

In a review of lung cancer patients' hospital charts, Greenberg concluded that socioeconomic as well as medical factors determined the patients' choice of treatment, which varied according to marital status, insurance coverage, and proximity to the treatment center. Patients were more likely to be treated surgically if they were married or had private medical insurance; patients without these factors were treated with radiation or chemotherapy. While the privately insured and married patients were treated more aggressively, they did not survive longer after diagnosis than patients treated with radiation or chemotherapy.[52]

Life Insurance and Cancer

Many persons with a cancer history complain of difficulty obtaining life insurance, although additional premiums can be structured to cover increased mortality anticipated by diseases such as cancer. Approximately 90% of life insurance applicants are offered standard insurance; 8%, rated insurance; and 2% are declined, according to a study by Elder.[28]

An individual with a cancer health history who does not receive a favorable response from an insurance company should seek out an insurance broker who can provide information on companies that are likely to evaluate applications realistically. In this way, it may be possible to obtain life insurance albeit at a higher premium and with a waiting period.

NEGOTIATING THE COMPLEX HEALTH CARE SYSTEM

Many cancer patients are uncomfortable with health professionals and persons of authority and they may feel lost in a medical milieu. They may understand little of what is occurring and may be too intimidated to question anything. Such patients do not view themselves as being part of the health care team but as having something done to them. These views reinforce a victim mentality.

The social worker is the team member who does not carry out any medical procedures and is trained to assess the patient's level of understanding and emotional reactions and thus can be an effective intermediary. The social worker can interpret the patient's uncertainties, misconceptions, and unvoiced concerns to the other health professionals and reassure and inform the patient. The social worker can be an effective force empowering patients to become active in their own behalf.

A generally accepted truism is that "hospitals are commonly regarded as an unpleasant place to be."[29] Hospitals create a depersonalized environment that forces patients to relinquish control over their daily lives. Health professionals have noted that patients cope with this depersonalizing loss of control by assuming "good patient" behavior or "bad patient" behavior. "Good patients" actually may be anxious or depressed to the point of helplessness, whereas "bad patients" may be exhibiting anger and reacting against what they perceive as arbitrary removals of freedom.[53] Neither of these behaviors is conducive to optimal medical management. Social workers can be helpful in encouraging patients to become better informed and more participatory in their care.

The effects of age bias, marital status, and gender are other factors inhibiting patient negotiation of the health care system.

A study by Greenberg and coworkers found that older women were less often treated aggressively for breast cancer than were younger women.[52] According to a study by Houts et al., at least 72% of patients who died of cancer in Pennsylvania experienced during their terminal phase at least one unmet need. Most frequently reported was assistance with activities of daily living. Other unmet needs of the terminally ill identified in the study were transportation, problems with medical staff, and insurance problems.[24]

Access to medical care appears to be easiest for middle-aged, employed, married persons and the most difficult for older, unmarried persons; persons with low incomes; persons with inadequate or no insurance; or patients in the final months of life. Social workers should be particularly vigilant in targeting these high-risk individuals for intervention.

CONCLUSION

Cancer can evoke powerful emotions and serious stresses that must be dealt with to avoid psychosocial morbidity and social disruption. It is possible for most patients and families to discover ways of successfully coping with this disease.

Many sources of social support and resources are important to the cancer patient's recovery. The presence of social supports aids all patients as they face the physical and emotional challenges associated with the threat to survival, value changes, and the demands on personal and social resources. Oncology social workers can provide much of that support and help to rally other sources of support for individuals faced with cancer.

While the field of oncology can be stressful, social workers witness the strength and courage of people facing adversity and are aware that minimal intervention on their part often can make an enormous difference to patients and their families. Understanding the common experiences of cancer enables social workers to shore up patients' personal strengths and sustain them as they struggle to successfully manage the cancer experience.

REFERENCES

1. Cordoba C, Cohen J. Problems of families with multiple cancers. *J Clin Oncol.* 1988;6:205-216.

2. *Cancer Facts and Figures, 1992*. Atlanta, Ga: American Cancer Society; 1992.

3. Fobair P, Cordoba C. Scope and magnitude of the cancer problem in psychosocial research. In: Cohen J, Cullen J, Martin R, eds. P*sychosocial Aspects of Cancer.* New York, NY: Raven Press; 1982: 9-31.

4. Koocher G, O'Malley J. *The Damocles Syndrome*. New York, NY: McGraw-Hill; 1981:114-119.

5. Yasko J, Greene P. Coping with problems related to cancer and cancer treatment. In: Holleb A, ed. *The American Cancer Society Cancer Book.* Garden City, NY: Doubleday and Co; 1986: 171-200.

6. Boyd N, Selby P, Sutherland N, Hogg S. Measurement of the clinical

status of patients with breast cancer: evidence for the validity of self-assessment with linear analogue scales. *J Clin Epidemiol.* 1988;41:243-260.

7. Cassileth B, Walsh W, Lusk E. Psychosocial correlates of cancer survival: a subsequent report 3-8 years after cancer diagnosis. *J Clin Oncol.* 1988;11:1753-1759.

8. Scott D, Eisendrath S. Dynamics of the recovery process following initial diagnosis of breast cancer. *J Psychosoc Oncol.* 1986;3:53-66.

9. Cassileth B, Lusk E, Bodenheimer B, Farber J, Jochimsen P, Morrin-Taylor B. Chemotherapeutic toxicity: the relationship between patient's pretreatment expectations and post-treatment results. *Am J Clin Oncol.* 1985;8:419-425.

10. Fobair P, Hoppe R, Bloom J, Cox R, Varghese A, Spiegel D. Psychosocial problems among survivors of Hodgkin's disease. *J Clin Oncol.* 1986;4:805-814.

11. Bloom J, Gorsky R, Fobair P, et al. Physical performance at work and at leisure: validation of a measure of biological energy in a sample of cancer survivors. *J Clin Epidemiol.* 1988;41:243-260.

12. Steinberg M, Juliano M, Wise L. Psychosocial outcome of lumpectomy vs. mastectomy in the treatment of breast cancer. *Am J Psychiatry.* 1985;142:34-39.

13. Mages N, Castro J, Fobair P, Hall J, Harrison I, Mendelsohn G, et al. Patterns of psychosocial response to cancer: can effective adaptation be predicted? *Int J Radiation Oncol Biol Phys.* 1981;7:385-392.

14. Taylor S, Lichtman R, Wood J, Bluming A, Dosik G, Leiborwitz R. Illness-related and treatment-related factors in psychological adjustment to breast cancer. *Cancer.* 1985;55:2506-2513.

15. Derogatis LR, Kourlesis SM. An approach to evaluation of sexual problems in the cancer patient. *CA.* 1981;31:46.

16. Cohen J, Cordoba C. Psychologic, social, and economic aspects of cancer. In: Nyhuys L, ed. *Surgery Annual,* 15. Norwalk, Conn: Appleton-Century-Crofts; 1983:99-112.

17. Anderson B, Turnquist D, LaPolla J, Turner D. Sexual functioning after treatment of in situ vulvar cancer: preliminary report. *Obstet Gynecol.* 1988;71:15-19.

18. Rieker P, Edbrill S, Garnick M. Curative testis cancer therapy: psychosocial sequelae. *J Clin Oncol.* 1985;3:1117-1126.

19. Schover L, Von Eschenbach A. Sexual and marital relationship after

radiotherapy for seminoma. *Urology.* 1986;27:117-123.
20. Bergman B, Damber J, Littbrand B, Sjogren K, Tomic R. Sexual function in prostate cancer patients treated with radiation therapy, chemotherapy, or estrogens. *Br J Urol.* 1984;56:64-69.
21. Cleeland C. The impact of pain on the patient with cancer. *Cancer.* 1984;54:2635-2641.
22. Holland J, Cullen L. New insights and attitudes. In: Holleb A, ed. *The American Cancer Society Cancer Book.* Garden City, NY: Doubleday and Co; 1986:3-14.
23. Greenleigh Associates. *Report on the social, economic, and psychological needs of cancer patients in California: major findings and implications.* San Francisco, Calif: American Cancer Society, California Division; 1979.
24. Houts P, Yasko J, Kahn B, Schelzel G, Marconi K. Unmet psychological, social, and economic needs of persons with cancer in Pennsylvania. *Cancer.* 1986;58:2355-2361.
25. Cassileth B, Lusk E, Brown L, Cross P, Walsh W, Hurwitz S. Factors associated with psychological distress in cancer patients. *Med Pediatric Oncol.* 1986;14:251-254.
26. Cella D, Tross S. Psychosocial adjustment to survival from Hodgkin's disease. *J Consult Clin Psychol.* 1986;54:616-622.
27. Lansky S, List M, Herrmann C, Ets-Hokin E, Das Gupta T, Wilbanks G, et al. Absence of major depressive disorder in female cancer patients. *J Clin Oncol.* 1985;3:1553-1560.
28. Elder W. An overview of life insurance and cancer. In: *Proceedings of Workshop on Employment, Insurance, and the Patient With Cancer.* New York, NY: American Cancer Society, Inc; 1987:27- 35.
29. Stahly G. Psychosocial aspects of the stigma of cancer: an overview. *J Psychosoc Oncol.* 1988;6:3-28.
30. Hahn R, Petitti D. Minnesota Multiphasic Personality Inventory-rated depression and the incidence of breast cancer. *Cancer.* 1988;61:845-848.
31. Joffres H, Reed D, Nomura A. Psychosocial processes and cancer incidence among Japanese men in Hawaii. *Am J Epidemiol.* 1985;121: 488-500.
32. Kaplan G, Reynolds P. Depression and cancer mortality and morbidity: prospective evidence for the Alameda County study. *J Behav Med.* 1988;11:1-13.

33. Mullan F. Seasons of survival: reflections of a physician with cancer. *N Engl J Med.* 1985;Vol 313: No 4:270-273.
34. Bloom J. Social support, accommodation to stress, and adjustment to breast cancer. *Soc Sci Med.* 1982;16:1329-1338.
35. Friedman L, Baer P, Nelson D, Lane M, Smith F, Dworkins R. Women with breast cancer: perception of family functioning and adjustment to illness. *Psychosoc Med.* 1988;50:529-540.
36. Northouse L. Social supports in patients' and husbands' adjustment to breast cancer. *Nurs Res.* 1988;37:91-95.
37. Weisman A. *Coping With Cancer.* New York, NY: McGraw- Hill; 1979.
38. Feldman F. The return to work: the question of workability. In: *Proceedings of Workshop on Employment, Insurance, and the Patient With Cancer.* New York, NY: American Cancer Society, Inc; 1987:27-35.
39. Barofsky G. *Work experiences and the cancer patient: problems and solutions.* Presented at Cancer Patients in the Workplace Symposium. American Cancer Society, Philadelphia Division, Inc; 1985.
40. Bergman B, Sorenson S. Return to work among patients with small cell lung cancer. *Eur J Respir Dis.* 1987;70:49-53.
41. Fobair P, Bloom J, Hoppe R, Varghese A, Cox R, Speigel D. Work patterns among long-term survivors of Hodgkins disease. In: Barofsky I, ed. *Work and Illness: The Cancer Patient.* New York, NY: Praeger, 1989; 95-115.
42. Mellette S. *The Cancer Patient At Work.* Atlanta, GA: The American Cancer Society, 1985; 4-17.
43. Crothers H. Health insurance: problems and solutions for people with cancer histories. In: *Proceedings of Fifth National Conference on Human Values and Cancer.* New York, NY: American Cancer Society, Inc; 1987:100-109.
44. Crothers H. Employment problems of cancer survivors: local problems and local solutions. In: *Proceedings of Workshop on Employment, Insurance, and the Patient With Cancer.* New York, NY: American Cancer Society, Inc; 1987:51-57.
45. Houts P, Yasko J, Simmonds M, Kahn I, Scheltel G, Marconi K, et al. A comparison of problems reported by persons with cancer and their same sex siblings. *J Clin Epidemiol.* 1988;41:875-881.
46. Hoffman B. Employment solutions. In: *Proceedings of Fifth National Conference on Human Values and Cancer.* New York, NY: Amer-

ican Cancer Society, Inc; 1987:93-99.
47. Holmes G, Baker A, Hassanein R, Bovee E, Mulvihill J, Meyers M, et al. The availability of insurance to long-term survivors of childhood cancer. *Cancer.* 1986;57:190-193.
48. Marshall-Cohen L. The Comprehensive Health Insurance Plan (CHIP): issues from the Illinois experience. In: *Proceedings of Workshop on Employment, Insurance, and the Patient With Cancer.* New York, NY: American Cancer Society, Inc; 1987:77-81.
49. Burton L, Zones J. *The incidence of insurance barriers and employment discrimination among Californians with a cancer health history in 1983: a projection.* Oakland, Calif; American Cancer Society, California Division; 1982.
50. Mor V. Work loss, insurance coverage, and financial burden among cancer patients. In: *Proceedings of Workshop on Employment, Insurance, and the Patient With Cancer.* New York, NY; American Cancer Society, Inc; 1987:5-10.
51. Greenwold, H. HMO membership copayment and initiation of care for cancer: a study of working adults. *Am J Public Health.* 1987;77: 461-466.
52. Greenberg E, Chute C, Stukel T, Baron J, Freeman D, Yates J, et al. Social and economic factors in the choice of lung cancer treatment. *N Engl J Med.* 1988;381:612.
53. Taylor S. Hospital patient behavior: preactance, helplessness, or control? *J Social Issues.* 1979;35:156-183.

SUGGESTED READINGS

American Cancer Society. *Cancer: Your Job, Insurance, and the Law.* No. 4585-PS. Atlanta, Ga; 1990.
Mullan F. *Vital Signs: A Young Doctor's Struggle With Cancer.* New York, NY: Farrar, Straus, Giroux; 1983.
Mullan F, Hoffman B, eds. *Charting the Journey: An Almanac of Practical Resources for Cancer Survivors.* A Consumer Report Book for National Coalition for Cancer Survivorship. Mount Vernon, NY: Consumers Union; 1990.
National Cancer Institute. *Facing Forward.* NIH publication No. 90-2424. Bethesda, Md: USPHS, National Cancer Institute; 1990.

PSYCHOSOCIAL TASKS THROUGHOUT THE CANCER EXPERIENCE

Grace Christ, DSW, CSW, ACSW

Current cancer treatment extends over time and proceeds through specific stages. Effective social work practice with cancer patients is based on understanding the individual and his or her unique experience relevant to the cancer diagnosis, in combination with aspects of the disease and the medical treatment process. Describing these stages and specifying the psychosocial tasks for patients in each stage offers the social worker a framework for assessing social and psychological needs, choosing comprehensive interventions to meet these needs, and identifying areas where new programs need to be developed.

The framework outlined here divides the cancer experience into the following stages:

- Diagnosis
- Initiation of treatment
- Effects of treatment
- Termination of treatment
- Normalization/fears of recurrence
- Advanced disease
- Research treatment
- Terminal illness
- Bereavement

Each stage will be described in some detail. The psychosocial tasks of each stage will be noted, and examples of related social work interventions will be discussed.

DIAGNOSIS

For all patients, the diagnostic process initiates a confrontation with the reality of one's mortality, even if the biopsy or test results prove to be negative. When a cancer is diagnosed, patients describe feeling shocked, stunned, and emotionally overwhelmed. They often say that life will never be the same; that is, they will always have a heightened sense of their own personal vulnerability.

Weisman and Worden identified the first 100 days following diagnosis as a period of acute distress for both patient and family. They labelled this period "existential plight."[1] This period has become even more stressful for patients who now often have to make choices about the treatment course, weighing risks and benefits of several options. Many patients attest to the special anxieties associated with making decisions at this time. Therefore, interventions need to be aimed at quickly reducing anxiety and distress in order to enable patients to integrate the information they need to make these vital treatment decisions.

Although patients need well-organized information about the steps in the diagnostic process, only a few seem able to make use of detailed written materials during this crisis period. Professionals are dealing with this problem by providing information to patients using other methods such as pictorial presentations, audio tapes, video tapes, and individual and group discussions with former patients and professionals. Clinical information needs to be provided by physicians, but emotional support can be provided by social workers and other professionals who assist patients in thinking through and discussing the information they have received.

An effective way to reduce anxiety is to help patients begin to develop a network of professionals, veteran patients, friends, organizations, and programs that can provide specific and ongoing support. During the course of illness, treatment, and rehabilitation, too often patients are left to cast about on their own to identify these important resources and services.

A social worker based at a large hospital, for example, may conduct group sessions to orient family members to the hospital system and medical procedures. Information about where to wait for the results of surgery; how to find out about visiting hours, housing, and parking; and what support services are available begins to restore a sense of control over the environment and helps to contain patient and family anxiety.

Patient volunteers may also attend these groups. These are recovered patients who have regained a good deal of their ability to function at their pre-illness level. They are trained to share their experiences effectively with other patients. These patient volunteers reduce family members' anxiety, as they demonstrate the potential to survive and continue living effectively.

The patient volunteers can provide information about the illness and treatment experience, describe the typical thoughts and feelings expressed by other cancer patients, and suggest useful ways to communicate about the distress caused by the experience. The information and the experience of talking with a recuperated patient can reassure families and therefore facilitate better understanding. This intervention can also serve to introduce families to professional staff who can make up an important part of their support network.

A veteran patient volunteer visit with a newly diagnosed patient is another effective intervention. Patients often will feel reassured by a discussion with another patient during the diagnosis stage. When appropriately trained and supervised, veteran patients who have completed their treatment and returned to normal life can be especially helpful to new patients. Their contact with the patient can rapidly instill a powerful feeling of optimism and hope. For example, a woman diagnosed with breast cancer left the hospital and returned to her job. She described herself as being in a state of disbelief that such a strong person as herself could be so vulnerable; she felt as though her life had ended. She was able to appear composed and in control until she closed her office door. Her secretary discovered her in tears. A friend who had breast cancer learned of the woman's plight and phoned to share her treatment experience and her return to normal living. The woman experienced an enormous sense of relief after the conversation.

While such patient contact can occur informally, social workers can ensure more comprehensive availability by developing a veteran patient program. These programs carefully select veteran patients appropriate for this work and provide ongoing training and supervision. This makes volunteers maximally effective in their communication with a broad range of patients and family members.

During the diagnosis stage, a patient must accomplish five psychosocial tasks. These are:

1. Coping with the realization of one's own mortality
2. Coping with overwhelming emotions that accompany the diagnostic process
3. Moving from denial of the reality of the disease to acceptance of information about the disease and its treatment
4. Making decisions about treatment
5. Building a network of individuals and services that can provide emotional, practical, and social supports throughout the disease and treatment process.

INITIATION OF TREATMENT

As treatment begins, patients require much more specific information. If this information is provided before treatment begins, the patient will feel less anxious and be better able to participate with the staff in meeting the treatment goals. Staff who provide information also demonstrate their competence, which is reassuring to patients and enables patients to become active participants in their own care.

Patients also benefit from advanced preparation for treatment side effects. For example, relaxation techniques to reduce nausea and vomiting due to chemotherapy are most effective if taught before the patient experiences these effects. Patients can purchase wigs in preparation for hair loss. They can adjust their diet to better accommodate nausea caused by chemotherapy or radiation, thus minimizing weight loss or weight gain. Patients can also be helped to develop a program for regular exercise during treatment that will improve their general health and comfort. Such advance preparations can enable patients to feel more in control of themselves, their bodies, and the treatment process.

When treatment begins, many patients experience a greater ability to control their emotions because they feel they are doing something active and effective to treat the disease. If they feel physically well, they are more likely to feel good. They are more likely to be emotionally upset only when they are physically distressed. However, this general lifting of mood is less likely with treatments such as chemotherapy that can cause many side effects that are difficult to control. Social workers can help patients understand the relationship between their physical condition and their emotions. Patients who otherwise may be frightened by unfamiliar mood variations are able to feel less anxious about mood changes when they understand them as normal reactions to illness and treatment stresses.

Family members also need guidance about ways to help the patient cope with the stress of treatment. At the same time, family members have concerns about their ability to fulfill their own ongoing responsibilities while the patient is being treated. If the patient is the major wage earner or emotional supporter of the family, the shift in functions among family members can be quite disruptive and stressful.

The psychosocial tasks for the patient beginning treatment will vary depending on whether the treatment is surgery, radiation, chemotherapy, or a combination of these. In general, the patient must:

1. Understand the treatment plan
2. Moderate distressed mood
3. Prepare for the management of the effects of treatment
4. Reorganize the family to accommodate treatment demands and offer support to the patient.

EFFECTS OF TREATMENT

Treatment side effects can have a profound impact on a patient's physical functioning and psychosocial well being, and can therefore adversely affect self-esteem. In reaction to these changes, patients may become ambivalent about continuing treatment and may fail to comply with treatment requirements or terminate treatment. A number of psychosocial interventions have proven effective in helping patients cope with the stresses of treatment side effects. They are described in the following paragraphs.

> Patient "role models" of effective coping with the rigor of treatment can inform and inspire patients. Patients who see and talk with someone who has been through chemotherapy, surgery, or radiation and who has returned to normal living may gain hope that their distress will be temporary and that they will be able to regain an acceptable quality of life.
>
> Financial and other practical assistance can help to mitigate the demands of treatment on a patient's day-to-day living. For example, patients are often demoralized by financial and physical dependence on family and friends for such things as transportation to a treatment facility and assistance with personal needs.

> Social workers can help patients be less dependent, which can increase self-esteem. Social workers can train patients in stress reduction, relaxation, and other behavioral techniques that are effective in helping individuals cope with nausea, vomiting, pain, discomfort, other physical symptoms, and the high levels of anxiety that may be a consequence of medical treatments.
>
> Patients can also benefit from specific strategies that help to improve appearance and physical functioning, thereby bolstering self-esteem and a sense of well being. For example, the Look Good, Feel Better Program sponsored by the American Cancer Society helps patients find ways to use cosmetics to improve their appearance during treatment. Social workers can direct patients toward learning exercise regimens that will increase their physical comfort, assist them in maintaining their weight, and improve their general sense of well being.

These interventions can be provided individually or in a group when the number of patients allows this. The group approach is more cost effective. Some social work departments have breast surgery rehabilitation groups, which generally attract a high percentage of patients who have breast surgery. The goals of such groups are to inform patients of the physical and psychological aspects of recovery from breast surgery and to assure them that many of their reactions and concerns are normal. Patients learn about universal experiences such as fears of recurrence, changes in body image, reluctance to communicate with others about the surgery, and problems with depression and other emotions. The patient volunteer presents positive coping strategies and encourages patients to become active participants in their physical and psychological rehabilitation.

Groups for patients undergoing adjuvant therapy, radiation therapy, and chemotherapy have been developed in many settings to help these patients cope with treatment-specific side effects. When groups cannot be used because of patients' geographic distance from the treatment center, social workers can provide the same information in individual counseling sessions and with the use of printed materials and audio and video tapes.

When faced with treatment side effects cancer patients must:

1. Rebuild self-esteem compromised by the loss of a body part, hair loss, and fatigue
2. Cope with feelings of ambivalence about treatment due to side effects
3. Develop ways to have some control over side effects
4. Incorporate the physical demands of treatment into ongoing personal and family life.

TERMINATION OF TREATMENT [2]

The stresses of this treatment stage have been recognized only recently as the number of cancer survivors has increased. Recovered patients have described a special anxiety related to completing treatment. The patient's reaction to the end of treatment termination will vary depending on the reason for treatment termination. For example, the treatment may have been successful in bringing about a remission, or the patient may have had toxic reactions and been unable to continue, or the patient may have completed the treatment but the disease was not arrested. When treatment was not effective, the patient confronts the physical and emotional challenge of advancing disease and the need to perhaps pursue another treatment such as a clinical trial. Even when treatment has clearly been successful, patients feel apprehensive about the decreased contact with medical staff and the return to normal living. Expectations of feeling optimistic and relieved may cause worries that intermittent acute anxiety reflects an abnormal reaction or is a sign of poor coping.

Family and friends often expect the individual to return to normal life quickly, not realizing that psychological and social recovery takes much longer than physical recovery. Patients must return to the personal and social demands they had prior to being diagnosed with cancer, but with a changed body and new psychological concerns. Survivors experience acute fears of disease recurrence without being on treatment. Cancer patients are aware of what they have lost while undergoing treatment and fear they have lost whatever competitive advantage they may have had in work, family, and social life. Physical deficits may cause persons to worry that their friends and colleagues may socially abandon them. This fear is unfortunately acute as our culture values going through a crisis unscathed. Thus, there may be little tolerance or support for the struggles of the recovering patient.

Social workers can help patients to learn that apprehension, fear, and disappointment are normal reactions to ending treatment. This is especially true with cancer, where patients are at risk for recurrence. It is important for staff to acknowledge patients' psychological needs and to suggest ways for them to continue maintaining their physical health and to develop an optimistic outlook. Patients who feel less anxious about their health are able to develop specific strategies for maintaining their health. After one year, most patients feel much more relaxed about their health. With time, survivors integrate the illness with past life experience and develop new goals and aspirations that take into account a new situation.

Veteran patients are especially helpful at this juncture. Someone who has been through the anxiety of treatment termination can be profoundly effective in validating the patient's experience and in providing hope for personal as well as physical recovery.

Patients at the termination of treatment can be helped by the presence of a continuing care program that recognizes the importance of needs for information and psychological and social affiliation. Such programs provide less intense, but appropriate and helpful, communication between the patient and the treating staff. Such programs can be implemented at a low cost relative to their value to patients and to the institution.

When the treatment is finished, the individual must:

1. Recognize and cope with fears of having less medical surveillance
2. Return to dealing with personal and work situations predating the cancer diagnosis
3. Adapt to remaining physical impairments and psychological stress
4. Change expectations of support from family and friends.

NORMALIZATION/FEARS OF RECURRENCE

Social and psychological rehabilitation is one of the most difficult challenges for cancer survivors and their families and friends.[3-8] Like treatment termination, the challenges of this stage have only recently been recognized. The powerful, life-threatening impact of having cancer makes re-entry into society, re-entry to pre-existing roles and responsibilities, and revision of personal and social expectations enormously difficult.[2]

Cancer survivors often are faced with a physical aftermath such as limits in sexual functioning, cognitive deficits, hair loss, or loss of a breast, a limb, or other organs.[9] The idea that cancer survivors can resume where they left off is not consistent with the experience of the overwhelming majority of survivors.[2] Instead, the illness often has created a major discontinuity in their lives that brings about lasting changes in the way they perceive themselves and their future.[9,10]

Losses from cancer may be physical as well as psychological and social. Regardless of the type of loss, the person will experience grief over that loss. Survivors often say they are aware of a loss of living time, especially young patients who feel a loss of "innocence" or a loss of their sense of immortality. Important personal relationships may also be lost. Social workers must be aware of the importance of a patient's task of acknowledging and expressing the anger and sadness that accompany such losses. As the following example illustrates, some patients make extraordinary efforts to normalize their lives, often trying to function better than ever in an effort to prove that they are recovered and perhaps to deny the changes.

> A 55-year-old woman underwent surgery to remove her shoulder due to osteosarcoma. She recovered well from the treatment, which resulted in loss of independent movement of her arm. She then made extraordinary efforts to keep a beautiful appearance, to be overly responsible for her two adult daughters, to continue work, and to compensate for painful and less gratifying sexual intercourse due to chronic vaginal dryness from her treatment. Exhausted and depressed, she finally sought help when both her parents died and she felt she could not take the time to mourn them. In her view, she had caused her family too much suffering already and she was struggling to protect them from her sadness.[2]

Another example shows how family and societal expectations may not match the reality of the patient's experience.

> One young man became increasingly depressed when he returned

to a brokerage training program after a year of therapy for Hodgkin's disease. His family was elated by his recovery and expected him to return immediately to his previous level of functioning. He, however, was deeply concerned about being a year behind his class, unsure of whether he could catch up, and upset by the changes in his appearance due to steroid treatment.

The fear of cancer recurrence is virtually universal among recovered patients. While there is some evidence that this concern diminishes over time as the individual remains disease free, the consensus is that it never disappears. Anxiety can be reactivated quickly by such events as follow-up visits to the doctor or the appearance of new (unrelated) symptoms. However, after one year, it does not usually interfere with the resumption of normal daily activities for most survivors. This anxiety may be generalized and create heightened concern about all physical functions and a preoccupation with one's body. One study of 104 cancer survivors who had completed treatment at least one year earlier found that the only significant differences between the recovered patients and controls were a lower sense of self-control and more general health worries in the patient group. Cancer survivors appear to experience a continuing sense of increased vulnerability and of living a precarious existence.

Cancer survivors are challenged to find ways to cope with this continuing sense of uncertainty. It is common to try to draw some reassurance from reaching certain benchmarks, such as the 5-year survival mark. Other survivors draw support from contact with other cancer survivors, either as members of patient-to-patient volunteer programs or patient self-help groups such as the National Coalition for Cancer Survivorship. Cancer survivors say this interaction affirms their success as survivors, provides role models for ways to cope with the stresses of the situation, and reduces feelings of social isolation.

Cancer survivors experience social stigma that is often the result of the ambiguity and fear that surround cancer in the public mind. Because society values the appearance of strength and certainty, cancer survivors, especially those engaged in competitive work, often fear that disclosure of their medical history will bar them from full social acceptance and participation.[2] This discrimination can be expressed very subtly and may affect the family as well.

> A 30-year-old businessman was very moved by the emotional support of his bank colleagues when his wife was diagnosed with a rare pelvic tumor. He was given flexible work time, a lenient schedule, and a sympathic ear from his colleagues. But when it became clear that his wife would survive, the man became increasingly aware of a change in his professional status. His employer suggested that he should only be assigned to positions in cities where sophisticated medical care was available. This would eliminate positions with better opportunities for advancement. Although grateful for the opportunity to care for his wife, he realized it would mean a major change in his career development.

One of the most troubling effects of discrimination is the difficulty cancer survivors have in obtaining health and life insurance. This often limits their employment opportunities because only very large companies can offer them commercial insurance. In addition, although they may be valued for their competence, they are often considered a risk in a management position. Both of these facts make it difficult for survivors to change jobs. Disclosure of the medical history may limit employment opportunities, but failure to give it could cause an individual to be fired if the history is discovered later.

After treatment, survivors may feel less attractive, may feel a diminished sense of self, may be angry at their bodies for having failed or betrayed them, and may feel a continuing sense of damage or vulnerability. A survivor must build a positive self-image that places the disease in perspective, affirm positive aspects of the self that may have been forgotten, and establish new goals and priorities that incorporate the disease and treatment experience.

It is also important for survivors to overcome feelings of helplessness and hopelessness in the face of a powerful disease and to identify ways to master aspects of the environment and experience that they can control. Patients often feel empowered as they work to maintain both physical and mental health, actively address discrimination, pursue new relationships, modify existing relationships that have been stressed by the crisis of illness, and establish new directions for their lives.

Survivors may also experience changes in close relationships. They often describe feelings of social isolation. Because of the experience, they may feel a sense of being different from others and awareness of their mortality and vulnerability. Reluctance to talk about the illness for fear of rejection can contribute to this sense of isolation. A primary goal of programs for cancer survivors is to help combat this sense of isolation and facilitate the development of open communication with others that will foster more satisfying interactions.

Having met the challenges of diagnosis and treatment, patients seek to normalize their lives, wanting to be as they were before and seeking to resolve any remaining problems that make them different. Patients become increasingly concerned about mitigating impairment, whether it is loss of a limb, loss of energy, loss of self-esteem, preoccupation with physical vulnerability, social barriers, or employment and insurance barriers. A patient's focus on the impairments that make him or her feel most abnormal may be misunderstood by health care staff as ungratefulness for having survived. It may also be misinterpreted as a misplaced priority. After all, a life has been saved and in comparison all else seems insignificant. But from the patient's perspective, it is natural to turn to solving problems related to physical and psychological rehabilitation.

Cancer survivors often say that the confrontation with their own mortality caused them to reassess their values and reorder priorities, which made them feel better about themselves. The usual tendency is toward more emphasis on humanistic values and less on materialistic goals. More value is placed on spending time with family and friends, maintaining health, and enjoying the present. In the aftermath of illness, some survivors become more assertive and willing to put their own needs first.

Social workers can develop programs to help survivors accommodate these changes. A cancer survivors' clinic, for example, could offer a range of services to meet psychosocial needs and foster the formation of a network of patients who are off treatment.

Such post-treatment programs may focus on individual counseling, but patients may be more responsive to education programs. Seminars serve as a powerful motivation for patients' participation. Components of a post-treatment program should include seminars on current treatments, health promotion, and innovative strategies for improving life after cancer; informal open house meetings where patients can share experiences and socialize with others who have had similar life experiences; ongoing group sessions focusing on problems participants are experiencing in adapting to physical and psychosocial changes following treatment; individual consultation for help with specific adjustment problems; or employment and insurance consultation.

At this stage, a person who has been successfully treated for cancer must:

1. Grieve losses
2. Cope with fears of recurrence
3. Cope with stigma
4. Build a positive self-image with a new sense of self
5. Develop a sense of competence, mastery, and control
6. Continue satisfying relationships
7. Regain a sense of normalcy
8. Integrate changes in values, goals, and priorities.

ADVANCED DISEASE

Patients often say that recurrence causes them to re-experience many of the overwhelming feelings they had at diagnosis, but with less hope for the outcome. Research on the psychosocial impact of recurrence, however, suggests that reactions vary depending on treatment options available and the new prognosis. For example, treatment for recurrent breast cancer can offer patients a good chance of having a number of years of survival and good functioning. On the other hand, patients with recurrent leukemia may have few treatment options. Because of the intensive treatments and an ambiguous future, the stress on the leukemia patient will be greater and more difficult to manage.

The reactions of both staff and patient to the progression of the disease may make communication about the new prognosis and treatment difficult for both patient and staff members. The patient is fearful and reluctant to enter aggressive treatment protocols again; the staff is disappointed and may feel a sense of personal and professional failure. It may be difficult for patients to understand the chances for effectiveness and quality of life implications of increasingly intensive treatment. Patients must make decisions about treatment, yet retain optimism and hopefulness. As at initial diagnosis, patients tend to become more discouraged and hopeless than is realistic. This is another time at which recovered patients can be helpful in providing encouragement to the patient and family.

Feelings of guilt or self-blame are common when cancer recurs because patients may wonder if they could have done something to improve their chances. Staff need to discuss these concerns so that patients can be realistic and relieve themselves of this unnecessary burden.

Finally, social workers must assist patients with financial and other practical problems that may arise when treatment must begin again. Some patients' experience will have prepared them for recurrence so that they are able to fall back on skills, knowledge, and supports that have already been developed. For other patients, recurrence is even more stressful than diagnosis because they are overwhelmingly discouraging by the treatment failure and find it hard to start again.

A patient whose cancer has recurred, or who has advanced disease, must:

1. Regain a life focus and time perspective appropriate to the changed prognosis
2. Process information and develop communication with the medical team about the new situation
3. Alleviate feeling of guilt or self-blame
4. Resolve practical problems related to beginning treatment again.

RESEARCH TREATMENT

Information about treatments such as bone marrow transplantation and investigational chemotherapy can be enormously complex and difficult for any lay person to understand. In addition, overwhelming anxiety and fear often limit a patient's ability to understand this complex information. Social workers can assist patients in developing an effective system for processing information needed for ongoing decision making. Treatment goals, possible side effects, financial costs of different options, and available support services are the types of information that must be clarified. A patient involved in a research protocol may continuously engage in a burden/benefit analysis for which clear and accurate information is required.

Although the quality-of-life impact of treatment regimens is important, such information is often not available in a form that allows patients to compare it with other treatments or with no treatment. Current research efforts are directed toward establishing a methodology that would allow the protocol's quality-of-life impact to be quantified. Thus, patients would have a better knowledge base for comparing research treatments and for deciding which is best for their own circumstances.

Patients may be ambivalent about continuing treatment when the risks and benefits are ambiguous. They may be unclear about how much control they will have once the decision is made to undergo research treatment. A crucial aim of psychosocial interventions is to enhance communication with the physician and the other team members so that the patient's questions and concerns are addressed quickly, thereby enhancing the patient's feeling of control over the process.

Patients, family members, and staff may have different views about how and when treatment should be given. This situation presents special difficulties when the patient is physically unable to make his or her own decisions or when the patient is a child. For example, the family may want to continue treatment when the physician and staff believe the burden/benefit ratio makes it unwise to do so. Often, this results when the families do not sufficiently understand the potential outcome of treatment. Another situation, especially in the case of a child, may arise when parents are opposed to the treatment because it violates family religious beliefs. In such cases federal and state laws provide guidelines for all professional staff to follow in making decisions. Extensive communication with the patient and family may be required to resolve differences. The social worker must take into account cultural backgrounds, knowledge, life experiences, family relationships, and psychological and mental states of patients and families when assisting with decision making.

Patients are challenged to maintain a hopeful attitude toward treatment outcome at a time when it is necessary to prepare themselves and their families for the possibility that treatment will not be effective. Physical symptoms and treatment effects are unpredictable and fluctuations can be emotionally stressful to patient, family, and staff trying to maintain a balanced attitude. A young child whose parent is ill may exhibit behavioral symptoms in reaction to the emotional stress caused by this ambiguous, demanding, and changing situation.

Finally, social workers assist in meeting patients' needs for help with the financial cost of maintaining themselves on research treatment. Some medical costs may not be covered by third-party reimbursement and out-of-pocket expenses related to patient care can be high. Such expenses include transportation to and from the treatment centers, additional parking and food and lodging costs, and additional caretakers in the home.

When disease advances and standard treatments are ineffective, the possibility of research treatment increasingly becomes an option for many individuals. For example, bone marrow transplantation may be considered for patients who are in remission as a way of prolonging the remission. Regardless of when in the course of illness a research treatment is initiated, the patient faces the following predictable tasks:[2]

1. Processing complex information about treatment options
2. Coping with ambivalence about continuing treatment with uncertain outcome
3. Resolving differences between family and staff about treatment decisions
4. Maintaining necessary hope while making realistic decisions and preparing for possible treatment failure
5. Solving practical and financial problems caused by ongoing treatment.

TERMINAL ILLNESS [2]

Patients coping with progressive illness that generally involves increasing symptoms and loss of function require more intensive interventions. Terminal illness can continue over a period of months rather than weeks, as was the case in the past. This extension taxes the ability of both patient and family to maintain a meaningful quality of life during the often arduous process of dying. Patients who are still engaged in life-focused tasks may not wish to confront death directly. Often, it is a struggle to find a balance between coping with symptoms and functional losses and coping with fears of death. Difficulty maintaining open communication in the midst of such emotional intensity is a common psychosocial problems that needs to be addressed during this stage.

Often, patients must make new treatment and care decisions similar to those made at earlier stages, but now they must also cope with physical decline. Decisions must be made about where, how, and what treatment will be administered. The benefits of prolonged survival must be weighed against treatment side effects. Increasingly, symptoms such as severe weight loss, energy loss, nausea, and pain are managed at home, often with limited home support services. Because insurance companies have come to view prolonged terminal illness as a chronic stage requiring nonreimbursable custodial care, reimbursement for necessary home care may be refused. Thus, patients may be forced to be hospitalized during the final stage of illness when they would prefer to die at home.

A recent survey of cancer patients asked to describe unmet needs during the advanced stages of the disease showed that 62% had at least one unmet practical need. Such needs included financial assistance; home care including skilled nursing care, personal care and household assistance; equipment; transportation; and emotional support and planning.[11]

This study also identified barriers to patients obtaining needed services, most commonly lack of information about available services and inability to negotiate the systems needed to obtain help. Social work interviewers also found that unmet needs frequently were the result of family members not being available for assistance. Social workers have come to recognize that family and friends can become overwhelmed by the increasingly complex and demanding requirements of caring for a seriously ill person. When caregivers have increasing difficulty coping with the patient's needs, patients and their families may need to locate formal services for assistance.

The course of the disease will vary, giving rise to sudden medical crises and creating changes in the types of home care needed. Or functioning may be eroded so gradually that a patient may be unaware of the extent of the changes. Discharge plans made immediately after hospitalization cannot always anticipate the patient's future needs. An outpatient is not as easily identified as requiring services and few screening mechanisms are in place for determining the resources that patients need at this stage.

A range of new interventions is being developed to enable oncology social workers to deal with the problems that have arisen in obtaining practical resources for cancer patients and in monitoring their care. A computer-automated telephone outreach system to assess the needs of chemotherapy outpatients for a range of practical services was studied at a large cancer center.[12]

The results of the study indicated that computer-automated surveys are likely to have broad-based acceptance among cancer outpatients and that outpatients are able to comply with instructions for completing the interview. In addition, patients who participated in this monthly monitoring system for three months had significantly fewer unmet needs than the comparison group of patients who received standard interventions. Research should continue to focus on developing methods that have the potential to provide a cost-effective, universal, and ongoing assessment of patients' needs that would facilitate timely intervention and efficient use of professional staff.

The oncology social worker helps patients contain anxiety about symptoms and functional losses by helping the patient maintain necessary, open communication with physicians, hospital staff, and other caregivers; encouraging control of pain and other symptoms with the use of hypnosis and other behavioral interventions; interpreting emotional reactions in the context of progressive disease; and maximizing existing home care resources and financial support.

At this stage, patients also need to clarify the meaning and significance of their lives. They wonder what the impact of their illness is on partners and families. They ask what their life is worth and ponder what they have contributed to family, friends, and society and how their efforts will continue after their death. Patients may also confront negative feelings such as guilt about smoking or other life-style behaviors that may have contributed to their cancer or anger and sadness about lost opportunities and lost potential. By helping patients to vent fears of separation and loss, sort out their concerns, and separate reality from their personal feelings and fears, the social worker can help relieve patients of these emotional burdens.

Groups can be effective in improving quality of life for patients with diseases such as breast cancer, where advanced disease can continue for months with relatively good functioning. In a study conducted by Spiegel and associates,[13] patients participating in groups experienced less pain, depression, and anxiety, and felt a greater sense of well being. In a later analysis, Speigel found that patients in these groups lived on average longer than patients in the control group who were not offered the group therapy. Further studies are needed in order to clarify the meaning of these findings. One area of investigation is to determine whether longer life can be attributed to improved self-care in nutrition, exercise, and compliance with treatment regimens.

Whether young or old, patients have responsibilities to children, partners, other family, friends, and colleagues. Mobilizing the patient, family, and significant others to plan for the future of the survivors is an important intervention. Completing tasks helps patients and family confront the reality of separation, provides them a sense of control over a devastating experience, and creates a sense of resolution and completion.

Specific tasks such as making out a will, contacting family, assisting with formal job termination in order to secure health and financial benefits, or prearranging a funeral are involved in this process. Interpersonal tasks such as repairing ruptured family relationships, working on resolving life-style and value differences, arranging foster care or adoption of children, or engaging a family member to carry on the patients' responsibilities after his or her death, may also need to be accomplished. Patients often experience relief after such plans are made and are better able to share feelings and thoughts about their condition.

An important new area of social work is the development of special programs and educational materials for children whose parent is dying of cancer. These interventions provide help during the bereavement period.

An individual in the terminal stages of an illness is challenged to :

1. Maintain a meaningful quality of life
2. Cope with deteriorating physical condition
3. Confront existential and spiritual issues
4. Plan for surviving members.

BEREAVEMENT

Bereavement services traditionally have focused on individuals working to master the tasks identified by Worden.[14] Many acute care centers are providing more comprehensive services to the family, a trend that reflects a greater awareness of the potential for social and psychological breakdown following a loss.

Several interventions for children who lose a sibling or a parent are being evaluated by formal research strategies. One such study examines the effectiveness of a parent guidance program for children who lose a parent to cancer. The intervention focuses on the quality of the surviving parent-child relationship, the parent-child communication following the loss, and the consistency and stability of the children's environment. The negative effects of prolonged or complicated grief reactions may be much more profound than had previously been understood. Bereavement counseling as part of the support program of acute care institutions offers the advantage of greater continuity of care to the family. These settings also may be able to address more individual needs. For example, young spouses may find it difficult to participate in community bereavement groups that are composed primarily of elderly spouses who have very different life tasks following the death of a spouse. However, if such services do not exist in acute care institutions, social workers can refer families to bereavement counseling through the American Cancer Society, local family service agencies, or bereavement counseling centers.

During the bereavement stage, social workers can assist the survivors as they strive to:

1. Accept the reality of the loss
2. Experience the pain of grief
3. Adjust to an environment that does not include the deceased
4. Withdraw emotional energy and reinvest it in another relationship.

SUMMARY

Cancer is a complex disease encompassing various stages. The needs of patients and families at each of these stages point to the continuity of care oncology social workers must provide. Optimally, continuity is best achieved by having the same person assist the patient and family. However, continuity can also be achieved if information and responsibilities are carefully transferred to different social workers.

The tasks are difficult, the work load is heavy, and the hours are often long, but few areas bring as much personal satisfaction to the social worker as work with cancer patients and their families.

REFERENCES

1. Weisman AD, Worden JW. The existential plight in cancer: significance of the first 100 days. *Int J Psychiatry Med.* 1976/77;1:1-15.
2. Christ G. Principles of oncology social work. In: Holleb EI, Fink DJ, Murphy GP, eds. *Clinical Oncology.* Atlanta, Ga: American Cancer Society; 1991:594-605.
3. Siegel K, Christ G. Psychosocial consequences of long-term survival

of Hodgkin's disease. In: Redman J, Lacker M, eds. *Hodgkin's disease: the Consequences of Survival.* Philadelphia, Pa: Lea and Feiberger; 1986.
4. Gotay CC. Quality of life among survivors of childhood cancer: a critical review and implications for intervention.
5. Tebbi CK, Mallon JC. Long-term psychosocial outcome among cancer amputees in adolescence and early adulthood. *J Psychosocial Oncol.* 1987;5.
6. Mellenette SJ, Franco PC. Psychosocial barriers to employment of the cancer survivor. *J Psychosocial Oncol.* 1987;5.
7. Teeter MA, Holmes GE, Holmes FF, et al. Decisions about marriage and family among survivors of childhood cancer. *J Psychosoc Oncol.* 1987;5.
8. Christ GH. Social consequences of the cancer experience. *Am J Pediatr Hematol Oncol.* 1987;9:84-88.
9. Fobair P, Hoppe RT, Bloom J, et al. Psychosocial problems among survivors of Hodgkin's disease. *J Clin Oncol.* 1986;4:805-814.
10. Cella DF, Tan C, Sullivan M, et al. Identifying survivors of pediatric Hodgkin's disease who need psychosocial intervention. *J Psychosoc Oncol.* 1987;5:1-3.
11. Houts P, Yasko J, Harvey H, et al. Unmet needs of persons with cancer in Pennsylvania during the period of terminal care. *Cancer.* 1988;62:627-634.
12. Siegel K, Mesagno FP, Chen JY, et al. Computerized telephone assessment of the needs of chemotherapy outpatients: a feasibility study. *Am J Clin Oncol.* 1989;28:561-569.
13. Spiegel D, Bloom J, Yalom G. Group support for patients with metastatic cancer. *Arch Gen Psychiatry.* 1981;38:527-533.
14. Worden JW. *Grief Counseling and Grief Therapy: A Handbook for the Mental Health Practitioner.* New York, NY: Springer Publishing Company; 1982.

SUGGESTED READINGS

Weisman AD, Worden JW. The existential plight in cancer: Significance of the first 100 days. *Int J Psychiatry Med.* 1976-77;1:1-15.
Worden JW. *Grief Counseling and Grief Therapy.* 2nd ed. New York, NY: Springer Publishing Company; 1991.

SOCIAL WORK SERVICES FOR ADULT CANCER PATIENTS AND THEIR FAMILIES

Diane Blum, MSW, ACSW

INTRODUCTION

Cancer patients and their families are found not only in medical and other health care settings, but in their homes, offices, schools, places of worship, and other community settings. Social workers, regardless of their practice setting, will be presented with people struggling with cancer's impact. Cancer is characterized by both acute and chronic phases. Social workers will be intervening during periods of acute stress and disorganization as well as providing services designed to have an impact on long-term quality of life.

Cancer differs from other chronic illnesses in that it evokes our deepest fears about death and questions related to the meaning of life. Although increasing numbers of patients are surviving cancer, about one-half will still die from it. The impact of this reality on patients and professional caregivers cannot be minimized. Since professionals struggle with the same existential issues as our patients, we can experience reluctance or ambivalence regarding involvement with this population. While our own feelings must certainly be addressed, social work with oncology patients offers significant opportunities to profoundly influence the quality of a family's experience with chronic illness. This potential to truly strengthen and enrich patient and family coping engages us in the practice of oncology social work.

This chapter will demonstrate that social work has a body of knowledge that clinicians bring to oncology patients wherever they are encountered. Skills such as active listening, providing support and education, setting priorities, enhancing communication, and mobilizing resources are applicable to any population. While cancer will certainly present problems to patients and families, these problems can be broken down into manageable parts and dealt with. Social work knowledge and skills will make a significant difference in how families learn to deal with the challenge of cancer and its treatment.

This chapter will describe methods to deliver social work services to cancer patients and their families to help them deal with the diverse medical, psychological, social, and educational aspects of this disease. Topics will include: screening and assessment methods; basic principles for developing interventions; a comprehensive service program of counseling, resource utilization and management, and educational interventions; and innovative service delivery and creative roles for the social worker.

SCREENING AND ASSESSMENT

Cancer patients are a diverse group whose pre-existing strengths and problems have significant impact on their abilities to cope with the disease process. Screening and assessment of individual psychosocial needs are crucial to developing a service plan that meets the specific concerns of patients and their families.

SCREENING

Since the 1970s, a body of social work literature has been developed describing screening mechanisms to determine who would benefit from social-work services. Patients who are identified as high risk by a variety of criteria are contacted and evaluated by a social worker at the time of hospital admission.[1,2,3] More recent studies are evaluating the effectiveness of preadmission screening, which allows the social worker to initiate a service plan before actual hospital admission.[4] Through both methods of screening, hospital-based workers can identify persons with cancer, chronic illness, or terminal illness as high-risk individuals who require routine assessment and intervention.

For the social worker who works exclusively with cancer patients, screening becomes more complicated; it may be impossible to routinely evaluate all patients. Cancer patients receive much of their care as outpatients; both patient volume and setting make universal screening difficult. There are several methods of screening cancer patients that allow for the identification of patients in need of social work services.

Universal Chart Screening

Universal chart screening involves routine screening of the demographic data and admission work-up recorded in inpatient and outpatient medical records. Factors such as age, marital status, insurance coverage, stage of disease, and type of treatment can all be indicators of high risk during the diagnosis and treatment of cancer.

> **Example:** A 35-year-old man, married and the father of two small children, with a new diagnosis of leukemia, and who lives two hours from the medical center, meets the criteria for a high-risk admission. The combination of aggressive treatment, predictable transportation and lodging problems, and having young children indicates that he will require social work services.

> **Example:** A 72-year-old man with recurrent colon cancer who lives alone following the death of his wife six months previous, meets the criteria for a high-risk admission. His recurrent disease and relatively new bereavement indicate that he will require social work services.

> **Example:** A 42-year-old single woman is being treated as an outpatient with adjuvant chemotherapy for her newly diagnosed breast cancer. The medical work-up indicates two psychiatric hospitalizations in the past eight years for depression. Although this patient probably will not require hospitalization for her chemotherapy, her prior psychiatric history puts her at high-risk for problems related to coping.

These examples indicate how routine chart screening targets patients who may benefit from counseling, education, and other services. In each social work setting, social workers can identify factors in the patient's environment that may cause the patient to be vulnerable to psychological and social problems. A systematic assessment of these factors by chart screening helps to identify these patients early in the treatment process. The obvious disadvantage of this screening method is that a review of demographic and medical data does not describe an individual patient's coping skills or resources outside of the immediate family. It also gives a picture of the patient at one particular point in time and does not predict adjustment to the disease over a period of months or years.

Multidisciplinary Rounds

A weekly conference attended by representatives of the various disciplines involved in the patient's health care is an excellent screening method. It is an opportunity for discussion by the team members who have interacted with the patient and for the social worker to discuss the characteristics that may make an individual at risk for psychosocial problems. The disadvantage of this method is well known to social workers in hospitals; that is, the difficulty of ensuring regular attendance by all members of the health care team. Multidisciplinary rounds that are sanctioned and approved by the various departmental administrations will be an effective format for setting priorities. Successful multidisciplinary rounds that have give-and-take among all the staff are both a cause and result of effective team functioning.[5]

Patient Self-Screening Tools

Several methods allow patients and family members to pinpoint their own needs. Cards containing checklists of needs can be distributed to patients through the admitting office or through any registration process. Patients can use checklists to describe their individual needs for help in areas such as transportation, home care, communicating with physicians, communicating with family members, or work concerns. Use of these cards also allows patients to become aware of social work services. The social worker's prompt follow-up response to requests for service is crucial to the success of this kind of screening.

The disadvantages of this method are that many patients do not take the time to complete a card; the cards must be collected and stored by a staff person in the medical facility; and the card describes needs at only one particular time. The card, however, can include information that tells the patient that social work services are available at any time. Such information should include the social worker's name and telephone number. (See Appendix A for a sample screening card.)

With computer technology, similar screening can be conducted by telephone. Siegel et al. describe a survey of 97 patients receiving chemotherapy in which a computer-automated telephone questioned patients about needs such as transportation, assistance with activities of daily living, and managing medical bills.[6] The authors present a persuasive case for such a telephone survey as a means of screening outpatients at different times, as well as for educating patients about social work services. If computer systems are not available, similar screening surveys can be conducted by telephone volunteers.

Any screening method may be compromised because the cancer-related problems generally confront the patient and family over an extended period of time, not just at a particular point. The effectiveness of an oncology social-work program will be realized only if the services are well publicized. Patients and the health-care staff must have knowledge about a social worker's function. Brochures, needs-assessment checklists, videotapes, and educational presentations all inform the patient about potential problems that may be alleviated by a social worker's intervention. As patients become knowledgeable about predictable problems and available services, they are helped in identifying their own needs and in seeking timely social-work intervention.

Assessment

Psychosocial assessment is the process by which the oncology social worker evaluates the particular needs of the cancer patient and those of the patient's family. Assessment involves a psychosocial history, a beginning treatment plan, and communication of needs and the plan to other health-care team members. The strength of social work lies in the ability of its practitioners to assess people within the context of their environment.[7] This is particularly crucial in oncology social work, where cancer has an impact on the patient not only in the medical setting, but also at home and at work. Social workers in a medical setting frequently must obtain psychosocial information in an environment of interruptions, space constraints, and lack of understanding of the social worker's role. Often, information is gathered from several sources. The oncology social worker must be flexible, must have knowledge of the disease process, and must possess an understanding of how illness and treatment can affect an individual's psychosocial well being.

Weisman presents seven questions that are excellent assessment tools for the social worker: [8]

1. What problems, if any, do you see this illness creating?
2. How do you plan to deal with them?

3. When faced with a problem you must do something about, what happens? What do you do?
4. How does it usually work out?
5. To whom do you turn to when you need help?
6. What has happened in the past when you've asked for help?
7. What kinds of problems usually tend to get you down or upset?

These questions elicit information about the patient's priorities; usual coping skills; and sources of support that is used to determine patients' concerns about treatment, work, insurance, family issues, and ability to cope. The answers are not always predictable. A patient, for example, may say that her major problem is her husband's recent stroke and her own diagnosis of cancer is something she must get through so she can resume care of her husband. A patient may identify a friend or coworker as a source of support rather than a family member. Answers may indicate that a person is not accustomed to talking about feelings or problems, or that professional help for problem-solving has typically been sought. The information gathered from this assessment process, along with the social worker's knowledge of the patient's cancer diagnosis and the method or methods that will be used to treat it, help the social worker to :

- Place the patient at a particular developmental stage
- Make a clinical prediction about how the patient and family will fare in this particular system
- Evaluate the priority that should be given to the patient in the context of many other referrals
- Evaluate what the particular health care system offers the patient and family
- Evaluate what resources are available outside of the setting to meet the needs of the patient and family.

Often, the oncology social worker may feel rushed in carrying out this evaluation and developing an intervention plan. Despite the short time that may be available for the process, the plan should be as specific as possible, describing steps that the social worker will undertake in assisting the patient and the family in dealing with their needs. The social worker's responsibility is to help other professionals understand how a patient will cope with the diagnosis and treatment and what interventions will be helpful to the patient.[9] An articulate assessment and a clear-cut plan enhance patient care and clarify the important role of the social worker on the oncology team.

BASIC PRINCIPLES OF ONCOLOGY SOCIAL WORK INTERVENTIONS

Social work services for cancer patients and their families must reflect the following principles:

- Social work interventions must be based on an understanding of the patient's specific cancer diagnosis and treatment plan, as well as the patient's emotional and social situation.
- Social work services for cancer patients and their families should be accessible. Most individuals with cancer need help during a time of crisis and they should be able to have direct access to a social worker.
- Oncology social work services are designed to help patients and their families feel more in control of a situation that predictably makes them feel helpless and out of control. Interventions should be focused on helping people cope with the medical, emotional, and social problems they encounter at different points in the cancer experience.
- The diverse population of cancer patients have needs that vary over time. A comprehensive program encompassing counseling services, resource utilization, and education will be most effective in meeting the changing needs.

UNDERSTANDING THE DISEASE

Cancer encompasses many different diseases and rapidly changing theories of treatment. The social worker may have difficulty keeping up with new information, but an understanding of concepts such as stage of disease, local versus systemic treatments, and risks and benefits of treatment is important. Vocabulary that describes specific cancers, the terms to explain dosages of chemotherapy and radiotherapy, and knowledge of diagnostic tests are also valuable to the social worker whose caseload includes cancer patients. The social worker who is knowledgeable about the treatment for and prognoses of specific types of cancer is better able to help patents set priorities, make choices, and experience a greater sense of control.

Learning about cancer can be accomplished in many ways. In a hospital setting, patient charts, multidisciplinary rounds, and conferences all provide the social worker with opportunities for understanding the disease. The social worker's participation in patient and family meetings in which medical information is being delivered is also quite useful. In a nonmedical setting learning may be more difficult, but opportunities are available. Excellent patient education and professional education materials produced by organizations such as The American Cancer Society, The National Cancer Institute, and the Leukemia Society of America may be useful learning tools. Interaction with physicians and nurses, field trips to hospices and day hospitals, and observations of procedures are all methods of learning medical information. The oncology social worker must be able to understand the reality of the patient's physical needs. Administrative staff involved in establishing social work services for cancer patients should also provide the social worker with opportunities for learning.

ACCESSIBILITY OF SERVICES

Most of the requests for oncology social work services stem from a person who is experiencing crisis. In 1967, Oppenheimer wrote, "The diagnosis of cancer with all of its implications can be counted on to precipitate a state of crisis of varying intensity and duration for nearly every patient."[10] More than 25 years later, social workers see many crisis points during the course of cancer. For example, moving away from treatment and intense medical scrutiny can be as unsettling as starting treatment. Certain individuals may cope effectively with cancer at first but will experience a crisis as they begin to deal with a side effect such as hair loss. Other patients and families may cope well with every need and demand until the patient requires intense physical care.

A social worker should be accessible when the patient experiences a crisis. Access to social work services can be built into well-designed assessment tools. Orientation sessions for new cancer patients are useful for letting patients and their families know about the availability of social work services. Geographic location of the social worker in relation to where patients are, a visible office, good telephone coverage, and continuity of care all work to make services available to the patient when they are needed.

Most social workers experience situations in which several days have elapsed between referral and follow-up, only to be told by the patient that the need had to be ignored or was taken care of unsatisfactorily. Rapid follow-up is important in oncology social work even if the social worker must perform a more extensive assessment later. A patient's problem may be lack of transportation home from the hospital or family members who desire information about chemotherapy. The social worker needs to connect quickly.

FOCUS ON COPING

Weisman states that "the existential event of cancer cannot be walled off from the rest of one's life."[8] Clinical experience with cancer patients has shown that the entire range of human behavior is reflected in individuals who develop this disease. Difficulties in relationships, developmental crises, pre-existing psychopathology, and the stresses of everyday living will manifest themselves in the ways people cope with cancer. A social work service framework must consider the patient in the context of his or her environment and prediagnosis strengths and problems. This perspective, combined with the social work philosophy of "starting where the client is," helps social workers develop a coherent service plan.

Social workers who ask patients about the problems the illness will create for them will gain important information about priorities at a time when patients are predictably feeling "out of control." Answers such as "I don't know how I'll pay my bills," "I'm terrified of feeling pain," or "I have no one to care for my children when I come for my chemotherapy," are representative responses. Social workers have the skills and knowledge to respond to these needs. They can also work with patients to help them feel a sense of control over a particular problem, and then move on to identify other difficult issues.

> **Example:** A 38-year-old single mother of two young children has a lung cancer diagnosis. She asks to see the social worker because of anticipated transportation problems when she begins chemotherapy the following week.

A psychosocial assessment revealed that transportation was the foremost immediate problem for the woman, who was reluctant to ask family members to transport her to treatment because she needs their help with child care. Although she was to receive disability benefits from her employer, because of the reduced income she felt she could not afford to pay for transportation by taxi. The social worker referred the woman to the local American Cancer Society office, which had a volunteer driver program that could provide for her transportation need for three out of her four visits per month. This assistance lessened her anxiety about getting to and from treatment. In the course of working out these logistics, the social worker and the woman discussed her reluctance to ask for help as well as her concerns about telling her children about her treatment and their reactions to her hair loss. The patient also expressed to the social worker her anger towards her ex-husband, who had not seen the children in over a month.

According to Weisman, "Good coping means: (1) good solutions for old problems; (2) adequate solutions for new problems; and (3) resourceful solutions for unexpected problems."[8] The woman had problems in all three areas and the social worker helped her to develop an adequate solution to a new problem.

Although the focus on coping and problem-solving allowed the woman to feel a greater sense of control, it did not encourage her to confront all the implications of her illness at one time. Rather, the process was one of separating out problems. The social worker assigned to this outpatient area was available to assist the patient over time in using her coping skills to deal with multiple problems.

Comprehensive Service Program

A comprehensive service program enables social workers to help patients by using a variety of interventions to address their needs. The following example continues the woman's story and shows how a comprehensive service program helped her deal with her specific problems.

Although the patient initiated the referral, her status as a single mother would have made her a candidate for screening anyway. Social work assessment revealed that she had recently learned she had lung cancer, had been recently divorced, and earned an income that met her family's needs but allowed no extras. The woman's parents, three siblings, and coworkers were very supportive as she dealt with the emotional impact of a life-threatening diagnosis and fears about the intensive chemotherapy. The assessment revealed the woman's financial stresses, concerns about her children's response to the illness and treatment, and injuries to her self-esteem as she recognized new limitations on her independence and unresolved issues regarding divorce.

The social worker predicted that these problems would be exacerbated as the woman underwent intensive chemotherapy, but that early intervention could alleviate some of the stress. The social worker drew upon a number of interventions to assist the patient. In addition to helping arrange for transportation, the social worker gave the woman brochures that described the process of chemotherapy and discussed children's reactions to parental cancer. The social worker told her client that the information generally has been helpful and that the woman should feel free to discuss their contents. The social worker also informed the woman of a weekly group meeting for chemotherapy patients that had helped people deal with treatment-related problems.

With these actions, the social worker helped the patient use community resources and also provided her with educational materials. By acknowledging the woman's concern about her children, the social worker began to develop a relationship that assisted both the patient and her family. As the woman underwent chemotherapy, she experienced stress over losing her hair, and expressed feelings of hopelessness about her future. The social worker used other interventions that met the patient's changing needs.

INTERVENTIONS

Social workers offer a range of social work services, or interventions, to cancer patients and their families. The choice of interventions depends on the particular needs and issues identified through screening or assessment. Some, such as referral to financial assistance programs, may occur only once. Others, such as counseling, may continue throughout treatment or be provided periodically around crisis points or when specific issues must be addressed, such as planning for discharge or for continuity of care in the patient's home community. Social work interventions are likely to be most effective when patients and health care professionals are knowledgeable about the comprehensive nature of needs and when the social worker is flexible and capable of using various clinical strategies.

INDIVIDUAL COUNSELING

Social workers in oncology spend considerable time with patients or family members discussing responses to the cancer diagnosis and problems created by it. At each stage of the disease, the patient may be faced with difficult decisions, with feelings of being overwhelmed, with communication problems at home or at work, or with personal feelings of helplessness and hopelessness. Injuries to self-esteem, feelings of dependence, and fear of pain and death are commonly experienced by the person with cancer. Through individual counseling the social worker can help the patient to focus on specific concerns and set priorities. An important part of the individual counseling session is that it may allow the person with cancer to express feelings and ideas that close family members have been unable or unwilling to hear or discuss. Many cancer patients feel that their psychological stress is a sign of weakness that makes them less competent in coping with cancer. Realistic reassurance and what social workers call universalization are important therapeutic techniques. The ability to tolerate and accept the patient's intense emotions (e.g., anger, hostility, bitterness, severe anxiety, profound sadness, depression) is an important therapeutic skill, especially when those emotions are associated with dying.

Frequently, individual counseling takes place in the patient's hospital room or in a clinic. Because of the potential for interruptions, it is important to try to create a sense of privacy, perhaps by drawing a curtain or positioning a chair. A contract of some kind is useful in helping the patient understand what can be accomplished by counseling. For example, an agreement to meet with the patient every day during a week of chemotherapy, or perhaps once a week for the person who is completing treatment, will clarify what the patient can expect of the social worker. The social worker must be sensitive to the fact that in a medical setting, patients and family members may be physically exhausted on a particular day and dealing with emotional issues may not be possible. When working with cancer patients, the social worker must be aware that time is short, whether limited by the setting or the patient's physical condition, and counseling needs to be tailored to the patient's energy and the progression of the illness. It is important to understand that traditional psychotherapy may not be appropriate for all settings. Counseling is provided to help patients and their families manage the problems associated with chronic illness. While this process is therapeutic, the goal of social work intervention more frequently is not intrapsychic change. In many settings, social workers have the qualifications to provide psychotherapy. When this is not the case, those social workers should be knowledgeable about clinicians who are capable of providing psychotherapy to meet the unique needs of cancer patients. Individual counseling in oncology social work has much to do with asking questions that elicit feelings and concerns and listening carefully to the patient's answers. The following are examples of specific questions:

- What is your understanding of what is happening?
- What are your ideas about what will happen over the next few days?
- How have you been feeling emotionally through all of this?
- How can I be helpful to you?

These questions encourage patients to describe what they are experiencing and allow them to express whatever feelings they are having. Useful responses by the social worker include:

- I see you look at things cheerfully. Do you ever have dark moments?
- The way you feel is so understandable. Many people in your situation express similar feelings.
- You have been through so much recently. It must be difficult for you.

Individual counseling sessions frequently elicit a sense of the patient's despair and the social worker, as well as the patient, can be overcome by feelings of sadness and futility. Trying to maintain or redefine hope is an important goal of social work counseling, however. Weisman states, "Hope is a prerequisite for good coping."[8] Billings explains that "Professional caretakers promote morale largely through an unspoken attitude that conveys an acceptance of the situation and an eagerness to do the best with it."[11] Oncology social workers have many resources for helping patients manage their despondency and distress and to feel that life is still worth living. Clinical experience teaches that most patients and families possess a natural inclination to retain hope. The following are general guidelines for structuring individual counseling for the oncology social worker:

- Choose a place to talk where there is some privacy
- Ask questions that are broad enough to elicit emotions
- Listen carefully to answers, paying specific attention to feelings, and observe nonverbal behavior
- Try to focus on one issue at a time
- Try to convey hope whenever possible, without creating unrealistic expectations
- Select interventions that are purposeful and address mutually agreed upon goals
- Review what has been discussed and set up a time for another contact.

GROUP COUNSELING

Purpose of Groups

Group counseling can be an effective social work intervention for cancer patients and their families. People with cancer frequently express a sense of isolation and feelings of being unprepared for coping with this unexpected crisis in their lives. The ability to meet others in similar circumstances, to share methods of coping, and to develop new relationships at a time of perceived isolation are all factors that encourage people to attend groups. Yalom describes groups as a way to help cancer patients feel useful and valuable to others during a period when they may question the worth of their own lives.[12, 13] Groups also play an important role in increasing the participant's knowledge of cancer and in offering specific techniques to deal with a complex health care system. Support groups, which are useful at all stages of the disease, focus on coping with, adaptation to, and living with cancer.

Group Structure

Support groups may be open-ended, with constantly changing membership, or they may be time-limited, from six to twelve sessions. The open-ended group is harder to lead because new members are constantly changing the group composition and there may be no opportunity for screening. The open-ended group, however, is sometimes the only practical format in inpatient settings or in communities with limited resources. The leader of the open-ended group must actively integrate new members into the group and prevent undue repetition. Both group formats may provide education using written materials, speakers, or videotapes. The educational component is useful in both recruiting members and in maintaining the interest of participants, who often come to the group looking for answers to questions.

Group Composition

Groups can be organized by stage of disease, diagnosis, age, or other common factors such as treatment modality. As a group becomes more homogenous, it becomes easier for the leader to focus its work. An 8-session group composed of people who have Hodgkin's disease, for example, will deal with a more consistent set of issues than a group made up of people with a range of diagnoses. Similarly, patients with newly diagnosed cancers may be reluctant to participate in a group with patients who have metastatic disease. Other groups may be developed on the basis of age or relationship to the person with cancer, for example, adult children or spouses of cancer patients. The social worker, however, may want to include a more diverse population in order to launch the group. Although this is a practical approach, particularly if the social worker is just beginning a group program, it is more difficult to focus a group with a diverse composition and to ensure that its members feel a sense of accomplishment.[14]

Starting a Group

Support groups provide a cost-effective service to a large number of patients and families. The start-up time of organizing a group and recruiting members is often lengthy, however, and months may pass before the social worker sees the time-saving advantages of a group. In their excellent practice handbook called *Cancer Support Groups,* Cordoba et al. describe the steps of a planning process that leads to the formation of a successful group:[15]

- Assessing the patient and family member population that is available. What are their interests and desires in relation to group experiences?
- Determining how many are interested in a group at the present time. Are there some who would form a nucleus for planning?
- Using this nucleus, involving members in selecting group goals together that fit real needs for mutual help, information, or discussion of issues and concerns. Goals need to be realistic and

appropriate, flowing from an understanding of where the participants are psychologically and physically.

- Dealing appropriately with staff and administration. Is the group concept acceptable to them? Include members of the system in the planning process; invite participation of other interested staff.
- Making provision for funds to sustain the group, including funds for refreshments, duplicating materials, and emergency transportation.
- Making sure that public relations and publicity are handled adequately. Collaborate with media representatives in the institution in contacting the media.
- Resolving logistical problems such as where and what time the group will meet and how participants will get there.
- Planning interventions in keeping with the goals selected for the group. Leaders must determine if they want a more informed patient group or a more self-reliant and socially supported group and decide what methods and techniques will lead toward these end results.
- Implementing the group program as planned or changing and modifying as new information and experience indicate.
- Building in an evaluation process of the group experience. Include a pretest and a post-test, and change with the times.

Even when following these steps, groups sometimes fail and the social worker will be faced with an empty room. Experience indicates that evaluation and inauguration of a new group, with particular emphasis on publicity and building support among other disciplines, will eventually lead to the formation of a successful group. Once one group is functioning well, it becomes easier to begin other groups.

Role of the Group Leader

Leading a cancer-related support group is a demanding, challenging experience. The leader always plays a vital role as the provider of support and guidance to all group members. In essence, the leader has the primary responsibility for setting the tone for the group, beginning with a screening interview and continuing throughout the group sessions.

Within the constraints of efficient use of staff, co-leadership of groups provides some advantages. If one leader is unavailable, the co-leader can provide continuity. It also enables the leaders to share and process emotionally difficult information more effectively. Co-leadership with other disciplines provides a blending of skills. For a population struggling with both the physical and emotional impact of illness, coleadership by a social worker and a nurse provides one such example.

The most important task for the group leader is to create a safe atmosphere in which members feel free to participate, without fear of judgment or ridicule. To accomplish this, leaders must be active forces in the group and consistently demonstrate, by verbal and nonverbal behaviors, that they can be trusted. No real work begins toward problem resolution until such a climate is established.

A number of common components are applicable and useful to group leaders.[16] The group leader:

- Sets the ground rules for the group, assuring members of confidentiality
- Takes an active part, particularly in creating a safe atmosphere for participation
- Starts in concert with members' needs and does not impose a preconceived agenda
- Initiates and stimulates discussion and allows common themes to emerge
- Provides appropriate educational materials and information on issues of concern
- Monitors the emotional pulse of the group; when painful topics continually are avoided, the leader may attempt to introduce them as needed
- Reinforces the predictability of feelings and places problems in a universal context whenever possible
- Works to instill hope for change and for improved quality of life for all group members
- Encourages networking of members outside the group for additional support and socialization
- Helps members join in discussions and strives to involve the more passive members as much as possible
- Leaves sufficient time to summarize the process at the end of the meeting
- Encourages reactions to the previous session at each successive meeting.

Evaluation

Making the decision to lead a group, plan it, gain the support of colleagues, recruit members, and finally, function as the leader for a period of time, can be difficult tasks. The completion of a group series that has had steady attendance and participation by members is exhilarating for the social worker and justifies the preparatory work. Objective evaluation of the group, however, is helpful in planning another group and also in convincing administration and other staff that groups are an appropriate intervention. Evaluation need not be complicated or elaborate, but should provide some objective measure. (See Appendix B for a sample evaluation questionnaire.)

FAMILY COUNSELING

Abrams[17] was an early pioneer in recognizing the effect of cancer on the entire family. Spouses, parents, children, and siblings are affected by the disease, particularly when it becomes a chronic illness, and the equilibrium of the family is disrupted for extended periods.

Family members frequently express concerns that are remarkably similar to those of the patient. These feelings include helplessness, confusion, and anger. Spouses and children may experience feelings of guilt because they may become impatient with the person who is sick. Grown children may have difficulty dealing with a parent's illness, especially if the relationship has been troubled. Also, caring for the cancer patient may burden a family financially and exhaust them physically. Family systems and/or its individual members may bring dysfunctional coping systems to the cancer experience. Social workers need to recognize these situations and tailor their expectations and interventions accordingly.

The following is an example of a situation in which family functioning is disturbed by the mother's cancer.

> **Example:** A 48-year-old woman with widespread cancer is the mother of three girls, ages 13,16, and 18, and the wife of a 50-year-old postal worker who works the night shift. Both parents individually report heavy drinking by the oldest daughter, school problems for the 16-year-old, and serious problems in managing household responsibilities. The patient and her husband both express to the social worker, but not to one another, their wish that

> "the illness would not drag on much longer" because they are exhausted. They have never discussed the prospect of the mother's death with the daughters.

This example demonstrates the need for comprehensive social work services. The family had home care needs, each parent expressed hopelessness and guilt, and the children were reported to be engaged in maladaptive behavior. The social worker used a variety of resources and interventions to help the family manage their difficult situation: holding counseling sessions with the parents and children, making the children aware of programs and materials for their specific needs, advocacy for the children in their schools, and offering homemaker assistance. The social worker also encouraged the couple to share their feelings about the wife's eventual death with one another and with their daughters. This helped to decrease the isolation each family member had experienced. Most significantly, by viewing the family as a unit and involving all of them in planning, the social worker offered them the opportunity to share their mutual distress and regain some of the closeness they had before the mother's illness.

Direct support of family members, both individually and in groups, is based on principles similar to those used to offer support to the patient. Specific educational programs and written materials for spouses, children, and parents are valuable in addressing and focusing attention on their particular needs. Resource utilization such as assistance in transportation and home care directly benefits family members and volunteer visitor programs offer the family a respite from care-giving. When providing support to the family, the social worker must view the family as a unit, communicate with them as an entity, and help them to communicate with one another.

BEHAVIORAL INTERVENTIONS

Social workers have successfully incorporated behavioral techniques into their repertoire of skills and have used these interventions with individual patients and in groups. In this era of shrinking health care resources, behavioral methodologies may represent more cost-efficient service delivery. Another advantage of these modalities is that patients are less dependent on the professional staff for help. They can be taught the techniques to use whenever they experience difficulty with emotional reactions to the illness or treatment.

Social workers may also use a relaxation or guided-imagery exercise as part of their group sessions. The group leader asks the members to concentrate on specific parts of the body and to relax each one until the whole body feels relaxed. Visualization of scenes or activities that are restful and create pleasurable thoughts is another technique that works well in groups. These exercises promote a sense of relaxation and calmness and allow the members to feel more in control of their feelings. Using this kind of imagery requires training, which can be accomplished by attending conferences or workshops on the subject.

Hypnosis, imagery, meditation, relaxation training, and music therapy have all been used in the management of cancer pain. Foley explains that "the major goal of these interventions is to promote an increased sense of control by reducing the hopelessness and helplessness that many patients with pain from cancer experience."[18] Knowledge of these techniques and skill in using them are helpful to the social worker on the multidisciplinary team. Training in hypnosis is required and is now available to the social worker in many settings. The ability to help patients control their pain and enhance their sense of control over the illness is a significant clinical intervention.[19]

Behavioral interventions have been shown to be effective for patients with aversive reactions to chemotherapy and fear of medical procedures. A number of investigators have studied and confirmed the effectiveness of hypnosis, progressive muscle relaxation training, and systematic desensitization with both adult and pediatric cancer patients who have been overwhelmed by anticipatory nausea and vomiting.[20] Similarly, these techniques have been used with patients who develop severe anxiety about procedures like bone marrow aspirations and spinal taps.

Behavioral techniques are now an established part of comprehensive cancer treatment. Patients, families, and other staff members are often appreciative of behavioral interventions that have a positive impact on the patient's behavior or mood. As social workers in oncology define and broaden their roles, behavioral techniques will continue to emerge as an area for training and professional activity.

Bereavement Counseling

Bereavement counseling is another intervention about which social workers should be knowledgeable.[21] The availability of such counseling will vary depending on the type of setting and staff resources. Hospice programs, for instance, are mandated to provide bereavement care if they are accredited by the Joint Commission for the Accreditation of Health Care Organizations (JCAHO). In settings such as comprehensive cancer centers, social work intervention for family members is often included in the package of available services. At the very least, social workers should be knowledgeable about community resources that offer bereavement care because of their knowledge about the effects of long-term illness and death upon survivors.

In dealing with an illness such as cancer, it is important to realize that grieving occurs at many points in the illness experience for both patients and their families. People often begin this experience grieving for the loss of predictability and certainty in their lives. There are losses of roles; losses caused by the treatment side effects, changes in body image, and ability to function normally; and a myriad of other experiences with which patients and their families must cope. Prior to the actual death, a process called anticipatory grief often occurs in which people face the simultaneous dilemma of remaining invested in the patient while preparing for the eventual loss. An understanding of this process and of those behaviors that are characteristic of both the acute and chronic grief experiences is important in assessing what kinds of services are necessary. Social workers should be knowledgeable about the differences between normal and abnormal grief, and grief and depression, so that they can educate families about what to expect.[22] Normally, people do not require mental health intervention to deal with serious loss. Most people, however, do not know what to expect in the immediate acute phase and in later stages of bereavement. Social workers can provide this kind of education and should take advantage of the many excellent resources available to educate themselves.[21,23,24]

In terms of services, individual bereavement counseling is becoming a luxury that many acute care hospitals are unable to provide. If this is the case, social work departments might want to develop a standard bereavement protocol designed to assess how a family is resolving its loss. For instance, routine telephone contacts at one, three, and six months might give the social worker enough information to determine whether bereavement is proceeding normally or if complications have arisen.[22] Hospitals or community agencies might experiment with time-limited bereavement support groups as a way of offering a more cost-efficient service. Groups are particularly helpful for the bereaved due to the normalization experience that occurs. Bereavement groups help to lessen the impact of patient loss and provide a way for families and staff to begin again.

RESOURCE UTILIZATION

For several decades, psychosocial researchers in oncology have studied the needs of cancer patients. Many of these studies have focused on psychological concerns, but more recent work has concentrated on what social workers refer to as concrete or practical needs. Mor et al. described a variety of needs among cancer patients, which they categorized as physical loss of mobility and pain; instrumental (daily home help, transportation, and shopping); and administrative (financial, finding help, paper work, and information). Cancer patients experience a constellation of needs, involving more than one category, and significant unmet needs can precipitate a family crisis.[25]

In studies carried out in Pennsylvania, Houts et al. estimated that 72% of people who died of cancer in Pennsylvania had at least one unmet need. The most common unmet need concerned help with activities of daily living, transportation, and obtaining home care. Houts' work demonstrates that the unmet needs increase as the cancer patient moves into the terminal stage of illness.[26]

The oncology social worker is well aware of the multiple needs of cancer patients and strives to meet them by providing direct practical help, offering information about resources and services, advocating for the patient within the medical system, and assisting in discharge planning. The social worker's goal is to help the patient and family identify and utilize existing resources as effectively as possible so that they can deal with the multiple stresses that cancer creates.

RESOURCES, INFORMATION, AND ADVOCACY

The cancer patient faces many potential needs: financial assistance, transportation, home care, prostheses, insurance coverage, and medical equipment. Interventions that focus on providing these services directly or information about them not only assist patients in obtaining the medical and nursing care they require but also have beneficial psychological and social impact. Examples might include:

- The provision of an attractive wig will have a positive impact on body image and self-esteem
- Facilitating the process of securing supplemental income fosters independence
- Assisting patients who need transportation to and from treatment relieves one burden of anxiety about the ability to comply with the regimen.

Oncology social workers must be knowledgeable about guidelines for assistance programs in various communities and must have an understanding of how laws are applied to the rights of cancer patients. Social workers also benefit from inservice training about entitlement and eligibility for community resources. Although maintaining current knowledge of resources is a challenge because of constant changes, such knowledge is a necessity if oncology social work services are to be effective. The worker may also consider developing lists of resources for distribution to patients. A guide to selecting an appropriate home care agency is very useful to patients. Even if specific names are not listed, patients can be offered general information about insurance reimbursement and what to expect from home care.

Oncology social workers may deal with situations in which resources do not exist or are not readily available to patients. Social workers who identify these situations may want to bring them to their supervisor and try to intervene directly to improve the system of service. Many communities, for example, have developed housing for patients and their families or have recruited a network of volunteer drivers to assist with transportation problems. The social worker can also initiate the production of written materials or videotapes that help patients function better in the health care system.

DISCHARGE PLANNING

Discharge planning is the process of putting advocacy, information programs, and direct service together. Hospital-based social workers who are responsible for discharge planning may assess the individual patient's needs, identify the most significant problems, and develop a treatment plan with the patient that uses family and community resources. Holden states that "discharge planning must be viewed as commencing with a psychosocial diagnosis of the patient at or immediately after admission, and as extending over the entire period of hospitalization. The event of discharge is simply the culmination of these earlier processes. Discharge planning is a clinical social work activity in which psychological, social, and concrete interventions are used together to develop a treatment plan that meets the needs of the patients." [27] Oncology social workers deal with the most frightening implications of cancer in the process of discharge planning. Patients facing extended care placement must confront their fears about dying; families may feel guilty about perceived abandonment of their loved ones. Therefore, the clinical skills are crucial to the development of workable discharge plans.

EDUCATION

Education is effective in helping cancer patients and their families understand the cancer diagnosis, use medical care effectively, and obtain access to the resources and entitlement of their community. Education has also been identified as a method to help patients cope psychologically with their cancer.[28,29] Blumberg[30] lists the following goals of cancer patient education:

- Adjusting to the course of the disease and developing ways to adjust activities and responsibilities of patients and families accordingly
- Achieving a sense of participation in and control over the care of one's body
- Preventing social isolation caused by the disease condition
- Normalizing life-style and interactions with others by developing increased coping and communication with family, friends, and fellow-workers
- Learning about resources to assist in paying for medical treatments and developing strategies to cope with other economic consequences of the illness.

The goals Blumberg describes are consistent with the goals of oncology social work. Information and knowledge enhance control, so educational interventions have direct effect on both the patient's and family's ability to cope with cancer. Education complements other interventions. Individual counseling includes helping the patient to learn about the disease and teaching communication skills. This knowledge can be imparted as part of the counseling process and supplemented by written materials. Group treatment, as well, can incorporate specific educational components using speakers, videotapes, and brochures. Highly structured groups with preplanned topics help patients deal with the enormous amount of information presented to them when they are treated for cancer. These educational groups are effective in both inpatient and outpatient settings.

Workshops that focus on topics such as coping with chemotherapy, communicating in the health care system, and using community resources can be offered to large numbers of people. Patients and families who are reluctant to attend a group or to use individual counseling may be comfortable participating in a workshop that has a didactic format. After specific information is presented, discussion groups offer the attenders an opportunity to present their own problems. This type of workshop helps individuals become more knowledgeable and also helps persons to realize that their questions and concerns are not unique to them.

Social workers in a multidisciplinary setting should consider organizing a workshop that includes medical, nursing, and social work topics. The social worker may direct the identification of topics, selection of an agenda, production of brochures, and recruitment of participants. Leadership in developing these workshops increases social work visibility among patients and other staff and serves to enhance the social work role.

Educational workshops focusing on cancer prevention and early detection are now offered in many communities. Establishing a community education program enables social workers in the hospital setting to develop interest in the social work services of their particular agencies and to have an impact on public health issues. Nutrition, stress management, smoking, early detection of breast cancer, and physician-patient communication are all areas of public concern and are appropriately presented at worksites and in senior centers. Community-based workshops, specifically at worksites, can generate income for a social work program.

PROGRAM DEVELOPMENT FOR SPECIAL POPULATIONS

Programs that address the psychosocial needs of particular patient populations offer social workers the opportunity to develop expertise in one area. Examples of programs implemented for targeted groups are those for people with HIV illness; Hispanics or other culturally specific groups; children who have a parent with cancer; and cancer survivors. Broad-based programs are also implemented for persons with a particular diagnosis such as leukemia or breast cancer, or for people at a particular life stage such as the elderly or young parents.

In order to develop such targeted programs, the social worker needs to embark on a process that is similar to that of beginning a group. A literature review, a needs assessment, multidisciplinary collaboration, development of goals and objectives, production of program-specific materials, and identification of evaluation tools are all integral parts of the process. Programs developed for special populations offer advantages both to the patients served and the social worker. With broad-based programs, a traditional service program can be identified. A social worker developing comprehensive services for breast cancer patients can focus the program on breast cancer from early detection through metastatic disease. Education about mammography, breast self-examination, and nutrition can be provided to healthy populations as part of a health-promotion effort. At the same time, women who have had breast cancer will also benefit from this education. One of the most difficult psychosocial problems associated with breast cancer is making decisions concerning initial treatment choices, chemotherapy, and reconstructive surgery. A program specific to breast cancer can include a structure for providing information and support for women making these choices. The social worker can also become expert in resources for women who are concerned about breast cancer or who have the disease.

At a time when social workers are increasingly encouraged to generate revenue either through foundation funding or direct patient reimbursement, specific providers of funds are interested in a discreet area of service that can be measured and described precisely. Carving out services that are traditionally offered by social workers and refocusing them for a specific population produces a clearly defined program that can be precisely conceptualized and evaluated.

Program development for targeted populations requires skills similar to those required to start a group, develop a volunteer program, or organize a transportation network. Social workers' expertise in dealing with complicated systems and functioning collaboratively enable them to lead the development of a comprehensive service program for a population with special needs.

EDUCATION, RESEARCH, AND CONSULTATION

Clinical social workers also have the opportunity to broaden their role and serve patients and families indirectly by:

- Teaching other health care professionals
- Initiating or participating in research studies
- Serving as consultants to social workers and others in the community who do not have expertise in psychosocial oncology.

TEACHING PROFESSIONALS

Service to patients and families is enhanced by the social worker's regular sharing of expertise in a multidisciplinary setting through informal contacts, written charts, and rounds. This expertise can also be extended to the education and training of other staff. Grand rounds, protocol conferences, inservice training sessions, and staff meetings are all potential forums in which social workers teach their colleagues. Additionally, to implement the teaching role, a social worker can propose particular training sessions on topics such as communication, management of side effects, pain, and sexual adjustment.

Social workers routinely assist patients in communicating with physicians and it is logical to use their knowledge to strengthen physician-patient communication. The social worker can use academic and clinical information to develop a presentation on this subject. The social worker can offer suggestions on how to deliver upsetting news in a way that allows the patient to maintain some hope and can also describe the variety of ways in which patients respond to bad news. The social worker can describe interventions for physicians or other health professionals to use in handling difficult situations such as dealing with a demanding or angry patient. A lecture or workshop presentation will formalize the social worker's teaching role and extend the professional influence of social work.[11, 31]

RESEARCH OPPORTUNITIES

Service to patients and families may also be improved by the clinical social worker's research efforts. The clinical social worker who is not trained in research may initiate a study or be an active participant in one. Social work research is implemented on a continuum of several different levels.[32] The first level is that of needs assessments or descriptive studies that can be ends in themselves or be used to proceed to more complicated research. Determining what needs are unmet is the initial step for a new service and is often the social worker's first experience with research. The needs assessment is generally carried out through the use of a questionnaire or an interview.

Many social workers are involved now in program evaluation, the second level of research. For example, if a social worker leads two groups, one with excellent attendance and one poorly attended, the social worker can evaluate different aspects of the groups. Questionnaires may be used to determine the patient satisfaction with each group or surveys may be conducted to determine perceived differences. Follow-up three months after a group ends may help the social worker determine the outcome of group participation.

The most complex level of research is hypothesis testing. A study is carried out in which the social worker's goal is to gain new knowledge. Social workers can carry out this kind of study with a specific population such as cancer patients in the workplace, or with patients who choose one medical treatment over another. Social workers are the principal investigators or coinvestigators in many such studies in psychosocial oncology.

Research allows social workers to develop objective databases that add credibility to clinical work. Research studies are used to generate new sources of income that, in turn, can support additional clinical positions. Social workers may find it useful to recognize the value of objectifying clinical work as a means to refine, improve, and extend the scope and effectiveness of clinical programs.

CONSULTATION

There are increasing opportunities for oncology social workers to share their expertise with professionals in community hospitals and agencies. Oncology social workers can develop the role of consultant by speaking at meetings and conferences and writing about their work. Areas of specialty, such as work with AIDS patients or expertise with groups enable social workers to present their knowledge to others. Consultation about specific clinical situations or program development are potential paths for clinical social workers to follow. Social workers can market their consultation skills informally or formally through mailings and advertisements, thus creating another means to bring in revenue for a clinical program. Such endeavors ultimately strengthen the quality of psychosocial care for cancer patients and their families.

SUMMARY

A broad range of social work services is necessary to address the many psychosocial concerns of cancer patients and their families. With knowledge, experience, and creativity, the social worker has a pivotal role in patient care. Social workers offer comprehensive services through effective screening; sound psychosocial assessment; carefully designed and implemented interventions such as individual, family, and group counseling; use of behavioral techniques; linkage to community resources; program development; assistance with bereavement; discharge planning; and consultation, teaching, and research.

Advances in treatment offer prolonged survival and mandate increased attention to the quality of that survival. This is the challenging arena in which social workers, with their expertise, can make a significant contribution in the health care setting as well as in the community.

APPENDIX A

EXAMPLE OF SCREENING CARD

At ____________________ Hospital, the Social Work Department is available to help patients and families with many different concerns and problems. Listed below are some of the services our social workers provide. Please check any that are of interest to you, and a social worker will contact you.

Please check:

_______ Assistance at home
_______ Counseling for patient and/or family members
_______ Transportation to and from hospital
_______ Financial concerns
_______ Housing
_______ Medical insurance
_______ Educational workshops for patients and families
_______ Informational booklets for patients and families
_______ Nutritional information (recipes, diets, meal preparation)
_______ Planning for the future

Your name____________________________ Telephone_____________

Doctor's name____________________________ Treatment time_______

Your social worker's name is______________________________________

The telephone number of your social worker is________________________

If you are interested in any of the services listed above at this time, please make a note of the social worker's name and telephone number so that we can be helpful to you at some later date. Please call us with any questions. Please leave this card with the receptionist.

APPENDIX B
GROUP EVALUATION

Group Leader: ____________________________________

Date:____

In an ongoing effort to improve our services, we evaluate each group series and invite comments from group members. All questionnaires are confidential and no names are requested.

Please take a few minutes to think about your group experience. Answer each question by placing a check next to the response that best applies to your experience in the group.

1. What made you decide to join this group?

____(a) To learn how to deal more effectively with my family member's illness

____(b) To acquire more information about cancer and its treatment

____(c) To talk with other people in a similar situation

____(d) To meet new people

____(e) To help others by offering information, suggestions, or support

____(f) Other (please explain)______________________________

____

2. What has been most helpful to you about the group?

____(a) Learning that others experience thoughts and feelings similiar to my own

____(b) Obtaining information about cancer and its treatment

____(c) Sharing my experiences and problems with other group members

____(d) Learning how to express my feelings

____(e) Belonging to and being a part of a group

____(f) Helping other group members

____(g) Obtaining suggestions and advice

____(h) Improving my communication skills

____(i) Other (please explain)______________________________

3. During the group discussions, which topics were most relevant to you?

____(a) Communicating with physicians
____(b) Making decisions about cancer treatment
____(c) Dealing with uncertainty about the illness
____(d) Dealing with feelings of guilt and anger
____(e) Dealing with life-style changes
____(f) Relationships with family and friends
____(g) Stress management
____(h) Financial planning
____(i) Concerns about the future
____(j) Other (please explain)________________________________

____

4. What were the most helpful methods used by the group leader?

____(a) Providing information
____(b) Offering direct suggestions
____(c) Encouraging general discussion
____(d) Providing written materials
____(e) Sharing anecdotes and examples
____(f) Encouraging role-playing
____(g) Drawing out thoughts and feelings
____(h) Other (please explain)________________________________

____

5. What aspects of the group would you suggest changing?

____(a) Number of group members
____(b) Number of group sessions
____(c) Group meeting room
____(d) Style of group leader
____(e) Mix of group members
____(f) Topics of group discussion
____(g) Time of day group was held
____(h) Other (please explain)________________________________

6. Which changes, if any, have you experienced as a result of your participation in this group?

____(a) A greater ability to reach out to others for help and support
____(b) An improvement in social responsibilities
____(c) An improvement in communications with others
____(d) An improvement in family relationships
____(e) A greater sense of self-confidence
____(f) An improved ability to adapt to changes in my life
____(g) An improvement in work relationships
____(h) A greater trust in groups and other people
____(i) Other (please specify)________________________________

____

7. If you had friends in a similar situation, would you recommend this group to them? Yes________ No_________
If not, why?____

____

8. What suggestions/additional comments do you have?

____

Thank you for your time and comments. We greatly appreciate your suggestions.

REFERENCES

1. Becker NE, Becker FW. Early identification of high social risk. *Health and Social Work.* 1986;11:26-35.

2. Berkman B, Rehr H, Rosenberg G. A social work department develops and tests a screening mechanism to identify high social risk situations. *Social Work in Health Care.* 1980;5:373-385.

3. Coulton C. Evaluating screening and early intervention: a puzzle with many pieces. *Social Work in Health Care.* 1988; 13:65-72.

4. Berkman B, Bedell D, Parker L, et al. Preadmission screening: an efficacy study. *Social Work in Health Care.* 1988;13:35-50.

5. Lowe JI, Herranen M. Conflict in teamwork: understanding roles and relationships. *Social Work in Health Care.* 1978;3:323-330.

6. Siegel K, Mesagno FP, Chen J, et al. Computerized telephone assessment of the "concrete" needs of chemotherapy outpatients: a feasibility study. *J Clin Oncol.* 1988;6:1760-1767.

7. Christ G. A psychosocial assessment framework for cancer patients and their families. *Health and Social Work.* 1983;8:57-63.

8. Weisman AD. *Coping With Cancer.* New York, NY: McGraw-Hill; 1979.

9. Mizrahi T, Abramson J. Sources of strain between physicians and social workers: implications for social workers in health care settings. *Social Work in Health Care.* 1985;10:33-51.

10. Oppenheimer J. Use of crisis intervention in casework with the cancer patient and his family. *Social Work.* 1967;44-52.

11. Billings JA. *Outpatient Management of Advanced Cancer.* Philadelphia, Pa: J.B. Lippincott; 1985.

12. Yalom ID. *The Theory and Practice of Group Psychotherapy.* New York, NY: Basic Books; 1975.

13. Yalom ID. *Existential Psychotherapy.* New York, NY: Basic Books; 1980.

14. Berger JM. Crisis intervention: a drop-in support group for cancer patients and their families. *Social Work in Health Care.* 1984;10:81-91.

15. Cordoba C, Shear MB, Fobair P, et al. Cancer support groups. *Practice Handbook.* California Division: American Cancer Society; 1984.

16. Coven E, Blum D. *Cancer Care Guide to Groups.* New York, NY: Cancer Care; 1988.

17. Abrams RD. *Not Alone With Cancer.* Springfield, Ill: Charles C. Thomas; 1974: 442.

18. Foley K. The treatment of cancer pain. *N Engl J Med.* 1985;313:84-95.
19. Spiegel D. The use of hypnosis in controlling cancer pain. *CA.* 1985;35:221-231.
20. Redd WH, Hendler CS. Behavioral medicine in comprehensive cancer treatment. *Clin Oncol.* 1983;1:3-17.
21. Worden JW. *Grief Counseling and Grief Therapy–A Handbook for the Mental Health Practitioner.* New York, NY: Springer Publishing Company; 1982.
22. Schneider J. Clinically significant differences between grief, pathological grief, and depression. *Patient Counseling and Health Education.*
23. Simos B. *A Time to Grieve: Loss as a Universal Human Experience.* New York, NY: Family Service Association of America; 1979.
24. Osterweis M, Soloman F, Green M, eds. *Bereavement Reactions, Consequences, and Care.* Washington, DC: National Academy Press; 1984.
25. Mor V, Guadagnoli E, Wool M. An examination of the concrete service of advanced cancer patients. *Psychosoc Oncol.* 1987;5:1-16.
26. Houts P, Yasko J, Harvey H, et al. Unmet needs of persons with cancer in Pennsylvania during the period of terminal care. *Cancer.* 1988;62:627-634.
27. Holden MO. Meeting diagnostic related group goals for elderly patients. *Health and Social Work.* 1989;14:13-21.
28. Meyerowitz BE, Watkins IK, Sparks FC. Psychosocial implications of adjuvant chemotherapy: a two-year follow-up. *Cancer.* 1983;52: 1541-1545.
29. Jacobs C, Ross R, Walker I, et al. Behavior of cancer patients: a randomized study of the effects of education and peer support groups. *Am J Clin Oncol.* 1983;6:347-352.
30. Blumberg B. *Adult Patient Education in Cancer.* Bethesda, Md: National Cancer Institute; 1983.
31. Blum R, Blum D. Psychosocial care of the cancer patient: guidelines for the physician. *J Psychosoc Oncol.* 1988; 6:119-135.
32. Glajchen M. Research principles for clinical social workers. Unpublished Manuscript, 1988.

SPECIAL POPULATIONS

Sue Cooper, MSW, CSW-ACP

Other chapters of this book have addressed the needs of special populations or groups of cancer patients and their families. Two groups, however, are discussed in greater detail in this chapter due to some unique characteristics. These special populations are 1) the elderly, and 2) persons with AIDS.

SPECIAL POPULATION: THE ELDERLY

Cancer has been identified as the most feared disease of an older population. Although age 65 is often recognized as the marker for "statistical aging" in the United States, one must be careful not to overgeneralize when addressing the needs of a group that can encompass several decades beyond age 65. Indeed, many 65-year-olds resemble 50-year-olds in their physical capability. Most people now consider the "old old" to be over age 75.

The risk of developing a malignancy increases with advancing age. Approximately 85% of all new cancer cases occur in persons over age 50, and half of all cancers occur after age 60. For older women, the more common malignancies are those of the colon, pancreas, rectum, urinary/bladder, and lung, with a somewhat lower incidence of ovarian and breast cancers. For older men, prostate cancer is the most common, followed by cancers of the colon, rectum, stomach, lung/bronchus, pancreas, and urinary/bladder.†

---

† *American Cancer Society. Proceedings of the National Workshop on Cancer Control and the Older Person. Atlanta, Ga: American Cancer Society; 1991.*

Social work intervention is especially critical for the aging population. It will continue to be an important aspect as this group grows in both number and longevity. A diagnosis of cancer in an elderly person occurs against a backdrop of a lifetime of coping and change, counterpoised by diminishing physical abilities resulting from the normal aging process and a variety of other illnesses with which the individual may be dealing. The elderly cancer patient's needs may be more concrete as the social worker helps him or her to maintain independence and control over day-to-day decisions. For someone on a limited fixed income, financial concerns may influence a decision to undergo high-cost treatment, especially if some costs will not be covered by Medicare, Medicaid, or other insurance.

In addition to advocating for the individual, the social worker may need to advocate for system changes. For example, more time may be needed to assist older persons. Physical surroundings may need to be made more accessible. The issues of an existing support system and the amount of support it is able to provide, as well as the patient's tolerance for accepting help, are particularly relevant to the older patient. Because a person without a viable support network is at higher risk for isolation and depression, the realities of the elderly patient's shrinking social network must be considered.

The special needs of an elderly person require a social worker who is willing to take the time necessary to establish a trusting relation, to use good communication skill including listening, and to be knowledgeable about community resources.

SPECIAL POPULATION: PERSONS WITH AIDS

Acquired immunodeficiency syndrome (AIDS) challenges all health care professionals, and the role of the social worker has never been more important than in dealing with this disease. Never before have psychosocial issues been identified and gaps in services been chronicled to the extent that has occurred with AIDS patients. The social, moral, economic, ethical, and legal implications of this disease are unparalleled in history.

AIDS is caused by the human immunodeficiency virus (HIV) that damages and/or destroys the immune system, thus making the infected person susceptible to opportunistic infections. Infections common in people with HIV include toxoplasmosis, *Pneumocystitis carinii* pneumonia, cytomegalovirus, and tuberculosis. These are caused by organisms that rarely cause the disease in people with normal immune systems but attack immunosuppressed patients. The virus is contained in semen and blood and is transmitted through sexual contact, sharing needles, prenatally from mother to fetus, and by transfusion of blood. (However, the cases of transmission through transfusions have been extremely small since testing of blood products began in 1985). Once infected, a person is capable of transmitting the virus. The incubation period can be from 2 to 10 years; the infected person, or carrier, can be asymptomatic during this time.

Oncology social workers have been closely involved in the care of AIDS patients since the disease was identified. Cancer centers saw many AIDS patients in the early 1980s because many were diagnosed with Kaposi's sarcoma (KS) or lymphomas–two malignancies closely associated with AIDS. Oncology social workers who dealt with issues of progressive disease and terminal illness with cancer patients found their training and expertise to be an extremely valuable foundation for work with AIDS patients. Cancer and AIDS share similarities, but the two diseases also are distinctly different.

Two issues highlight these differences: choice of behavior and contagion. Having sexual encounters and sharing needles are choices. Social work tenets of self-determination and nonjudgmental attitudes are essential in working with AIDS patients. A social worker must be willing to separate his or her personal, emotional response from professional responsibility to deliver care.

The second issue is fear of contagion. It is reasonable to be fearful of a contagious disease. The first step is to acknowledge the fear and the next step is to be sufficiently educated to alleviate this fear and understand the disease process. The virus is not transmitted by casual contact–people do not get AIDS by touching a patient, from saliva, sweat, tears, urine, a kiss, a hug, a telephone, a toilet seat, or a mosquito bite. Without proper education, fear can be a real barrier to effective care.

These two issues are especially important for social workers whose clients are AIDS patients. Social workers should be certain they are comfortable enough with these issues before working with AIDS patients to make sure that prejudices or biases are not thinly veiled and that fear of contagion is not a burden.When the issues are not resolved, effective casework is impossible and early burnout is predictable.

Who are the patients? The virus, once thought to have gender preference for homosexual men, now crosses not just sexual barriers but socioeconomic, age, race, ethnic, and professional barriers as well. The majority of AIDS patients are homosexual or bisexual men and intravenous drug users, but the incidence among heterosexual men and women and children is growing. (Children's issues will not be discussed in this section, as there are few incidences of AIDS-related malignancies in the pediatric population).[1] The issues relevant to these groups are listed in Table 1.[2]

HIV INFECTION/AIDS AS A PROCESS

Oncology social workers will more than likely see patients in cancer centers who are diagnosed with Kaposi's sarcoma or lymphomas. Approximately 9% of all AIDS patients have been reported to have KS.[3] Because of the chronicity of this disease, the patient population will be seen many times. Therefore, it is important to social workers to conceptualize care as a process and to identify the psychosocial issues that have an impact on the patient and family.

EARLY STAGE

HIV infection's progression to full-blown AIDS follows a very individual course. That is, a patient may start to have nagging symptoms that will escalate over time. Conversely, a presenting symptom may be the appearance of a KS lesion or a bout of *Pneumocystis carinii* pneumonia, an opportunistic infection rare in persons with an intact immune system. A diagnosis of KS, lymphoma, or an opportunistic infection will automatically move the patient into full-blown AIDS. Issues of concern at this stage are discussed in the following sections.

Confidentiality

In the early stage of the disease, issues of confidentiality are extremely important. Discrimination against HIV-infected people has occurred in the work place; with health insurance, housing, and social services; and in many other areas. Patients may not even want their families to know the diagnosis. It is essential that the social worker be aware of who is to know what information.

Table 1
ISSUES RELEVANT TO GROUPS OF PERSONS WITH AIDS

Homosexual clientele
Family support or lack thereof
Awareness of life-style
Confidentiality
Financial resources
Employment
Physical deterioration/appearance
Independence/dependence
Legal issues (partner vs. legal next of kin)
Spiritual strength/conflict
Isolation and rejection
Negative societal response

IV drug user clientele
Family support or lack thereof
Awareness of life-style
Confidentiality
Financial resources
Physical deterioration/appearance
Addictive personality and behavior rendering this group less likely to take responsibility for individual actions
Increased probability of bearing children infected with HIV
Increased exposure to HIV due to multiple high-risk behaviors
Isolation and rejection
Negative societal response

Heterosexual clientele
Difficulty sharing diagnosis with family
Confidentiality
Continuing employment
Disclosure of past risk behaviors (i.e., infidelity, bisexual encounters, IV drug use)
Spiritual strengths/conflicts
Isolation and rejection
Negative societal response

Denial

Almost anyone who has a life-threatening illness diagnosed will go through periods of denial because the task of coping with everything at once is overwhelming. Some denial is appropriate as a coping mechanism to allow a person to gradually sort out the implications of the diagnosis. Sensitive, honest discussion between patient and social worker can facilitate movement toward accepting the reality of the situation.

Appearance of KS Lesions

Although not all patients develop KS (a cancer or tumor of the blood and/or lymph vessel cells), those who do feel "branded" by the lesions because they often appear on the face, arms, neck, and trunk. Decisions must be made whether to begin chemotherapy or radiation; to continue taking zidovudine (AZT); to decide how to deal with work-related problems of being on sick leave and feelings of rejection; and so forth. These issues are more concrete in nature but still require sensitive handling.

Psychosocial Issues

Feelings of anger, guilt, and shame are ongoing issues, as are concerns about body image and intimacy. AIDS patients are usually young and have not considered death in the near term. However, contemplating one's own death usually begins in the early stage. Issues of finances and access to health care may have a somewhat different impact on the patient, depending upon sexual orientation or intravenous (IV) drug use history.

Education

At the time of diagnosis, every patient needs to be educated about the disease, to understand its chronic nature and its course, and to realize that early diagnosis does not mean immediate death. The patient should clearly understand modes of transmission so that steps can be taken to avoid infecting others. Safer sexual practice should be clearly defined and IV drug users should understand the risks of needle sharing. Heterosexuals should be educated and counseled about having children in light of the high risk of infecting the fetus. All education must be culturally sensitive and language specific. The goals for the social worker during the early stage are listed in Table 2.

Table 2
EARLY STAGE GOALS FOR SOCIAL WORKER

Establish relationship
Understand roles
Deal with psychosocial issues
Be active listener
Understand disease process
Know facts about testing, transmission, and safer sex
Be an educator

MIDDLE STAGE

As the disease progresses, a wasting syndrome characterized by loss of weight, fatigue, weakness, and possible neuropathy caused by infections or chemotherapy is easy to see in patients. Symptoms of AIDS dementia may appear and disrupt the patient's daily activities. Incidences of opportunistic infections may necessitate additional hospitalizations. At this point, the deterioration of health may signal that the patient is no longer able to work. Work-related issues then become a significant focus. These problem areas challenge the patient, family, significant others, and the social worker.

Lymphomas and Opportunistic Infections

Different forms of lymphomas (cancer of the lymphoid tissue) can appear as the disease progresses and further compromise the patient's health. Also, the longer a patient lives, bouts of opportunistic infections will increase. The patient's ability to regain strength and energy is minimal and home care becomes very important. Most antibiotics and blood transfusions can be administered at home. Those patients who have adequate insurance coverage may realize great savings by having treatments administered at home or on an outpatient basis. However, those patients dependent upon treatment in the public sector must remain hospitalized to get the drug therapy they need.

AIDS Dementia

The HIV virus is attracted to cells of the central nervous system and AIDS dementia (mental deterioration) is prevalent in a large percentage of AIDS patients. Symptoms of cognitive impairment include memory loss, lack of concentration, mental slowing, or confusion. Behavioral symptoms include apathy, withdrawal, depression, agitation, or confusion. Motor symptoms include unsteady gait, bilateral leg weakness, loss of coordination, impaired handwriting, and tremors. [4] Often, social workers are the first health care professionals to suspect or pinpoint symptoms of dementia. Patients may be referred to the social worker for their depression and psychotherapy when in fact the problem is AIDS dementia and psychotherapy is of little use. The patients are often painfully aware of their mental impairment. Many patients taking AZT have found their symptoms have improved when on the drug.

Work-Related Issues

It is important for psychological, financial, and insurance reasons for persons with AIDS to work as long as possible. However, when work is no longer possible, steps must be taken to ensure care. The social worker must be cognizant of the COBRA law, Supplemental Security income, and Social Security Disability guidelines, Medicaid and Medicare regulations, and local agencies that provide assistance.

Nontraditional Treatment

Few successful treatment modalities and research drug trials are available against AIDS, so patients often consider nontraditional treatments such as diets, vitamin therapy, and immune modulation. Patients usually confide to their social worker that they are considering and/or trying these treatments. The social worker can play a valuable role in listening, reality testing, and sorting out options. If the patient continues these treatments, it is essential that the primary physician is aware of what the patient is doing.

Legal Concerns

As the patient's health declines, legal concerns must be discussed. Does the gay patient understand who would make medical decisions for him if he were unable to do so? Who has guardianship of a single woman's child? Does the patient have a power-of-attorney, advance directive, health care proxy, living will, or a general will? These sensitive but vital issues must be discussed when the patient is mentally and emotionally able to make the best decisions. Most patients have probably thought of these issues so the social worker's role is usually not to introduce these issues but to facilitate the patient's resolution of them.

The goals for the social worker in the middle stage are listed in Table 3.

Table 3
MIDDLE STAGE GOALS FOR SOCIAL WORKER

Increase trusting relationship
Deal with psychosocial issues, especially loss of control
Management of AIDS dementia
Develop good discharge planning skills
Attention to legal concerns
Make referrals to support groups
Be aware of transference and countertransference

END STAGE

Most AIDS patients are aware they have a life-threatening illness. The death of friends because of AIDS and the progressive nature of the illness have given persons with AIDS time to contemplate their own death. Because of this, AIDS patients as a group may be more prepared to die than others. Issues to clarify are discussed in the following sections.

Choices

Where does the patient want to be–at home or in a hospital? If the choice is home, can a caretaker be there? Is nursing care available? Is a respite team involved? Can medication be administered? Will the patient be comfortable? If in a hospital, does the setting accommodate the needs of the patient, partner, and/or family? Is the clergy alerted? How is the caregiving team dealing with this patient? Does the patient want to be at a hospital? Is one available?

Intubation, Respirators, No Code

As for any chronically ill patient, these issues should be discussed long before the need arises. Patients have the right to participate in making the decisions about these procedures and the social worker's responsibility is to make sure people have correct information on which to base a decision. Many patients do *not* want these "heroic" procedures done, but many patients do. Whichever choice is made must be documented. Open-ended questions such as "Have you thought about how you feel about respirators?" can help the social worker and patient discuss this issue. The social worker who has a trusting relationship with the patient is often the person who can talk about choices and can facilitate a meaningful conversation between patient and physician.

Saying Goodbye

Part of dying is saying goodbye. This closure, or saying goodbye, can be done in many different ways–verbally, with eye contact, by touching, with parables, or even with hand signals. The dying patient needs to say goodbye to loved ones, friends, and staff. Professional staff can help to make sure that this final act of taking care of unfinished business is allowed to happen. The goals for the social worker in the end stage are listed in Table 4.

Table 4
END STAGE GOALS FOR SOCIAL WORKER

Be able to face reality of death with patient
Clarify options and choices
Communicate patient's choices to staff, partner, and family
Be supportive of caregivers
Monitor interactions of traditional and nontraditional families
Say goodbye
Make referrals to support groups, counseling, or other services for caregivers
Provide bereavement care for family, partner, and friends

FAMILIES

The AIDS patient may be part of a traditional or nontraditional family; the latter might include the patient's partner and/or close friends. Either family may be supportive or nonsupportive. Barriers to support can be the fear of contagion as well as the stigma of AIDS. Because the patient population is relatively young, parents are often dealing with the death of their child. This is an event most parents are ill-prepared to deal with as parents expect to die before their children. It may be physically difficult for older parents to assume the caregiver role. It may be demeaning to the patient to need the parents in the caregiver role. Issues of acceptance, secret keeping, morals, and religion can complicate family relations if the patient is gay.

For some patients, the nontraditional family may be a stronger unit because it usually consists of persons living together who care about one another who are accepting of life-style and share a similar value system. However, the nontraditional family is not a legal entity and this raises a special concern. Legal steps can be taken to give certain powers to individuals via power-of-attorney, if desired by the patient. This issue becomes a vital concern during consideration of treatment modalities, information giving, and decision making. Staff perception of the nontraditional family is also important because biases and behaviors that contradict an individual's own value system can easily be interwoven into the delivery of care. The social worker needs to be alert to this possibility and take appropriate steps to correct this situation if it arises.

When traditional and nontraditional families can function together, it can bring a sense of relief to the patient. Both units can be very supportive of the patient and each other, particularly when good communication is fostered.

CANCER PATIENTS INFECTED WITH HIV THROUGH TRANSFUSIONS

Some cancer survivors are being diagnosed with HIV infection/or AIDS as a result of multiple blood transfusions received while undergoing cancer therapy, especially if blood products were given prior to 1985.

Understandably, individuals in this group feel frustrated and angry at having survived cancer only to have been infected through the process that helped save their lives. Additionally, physicians and staff feel a great deal of anger and guilt for either having prescribed the transfusion or administered it.

AIDS/DRUG ABUSE DUAL DIAGNOSIS

The coexistence of AIDS and drug abuse is almost overwhelming due to the social stigma attached to both. Treatment modalities and resources are limited for this patient population that encompasses women, male and female prostitutes, runaways, and adolescents. Infected women will ultimately result in more pediatric cases. Patients in this group usually seek medical care in the later stages of the disease and find drug dependency to be a more pressing issue than AIDS. For the most part, the social worker's task is to locate resources available to meet the needs of patients who are both drug dependent and dying of AIDS.

RESOURCES AND INFORMATION

Table 5 lists resources and information needs that are essential to the beginning social worker who will be working with AIDS patients.

Table 5
PREPARING FOR WORK WITH AIDS PATIENTS

Resources:
Testing sites
City, county, state AIDS programs/agencies
AIDS organizations
Respite teams
Hospice groups
Visiting Nurse Association, home health agencies
American Cancer Society
Support groups

Information:
CDC definition of AIDS
Symptoms of AIDS
Confidentiality policy of hospital
Testing facts
Blood supply facts
Supplemental Security Income information
Social Security Disability information
COBRA law information

REFERENCES

1. Centers for Disease Control. AIDS and women in the U.S., 1981-1988. *MMWR.* 1989; 38:229-2336.

2. Cooper S, Weil J. Developing AIDS inpatient and outpatient services. In: Blanchet K, ed. *AIDS: A Health Care Management Response.* Rockville, Md: Aspen Press; 1988:120-121.

3. Centers for Disease Control. *MMWR.* 1989.

4. Bocellari A. The early manifestation of AIDS dementia. Adapted from: Navia and Price. *Ann Psychiatr.* 1986;16:158-166.

SUGGESTED READINGS

Suggested readings and resources for the social worker who will be caring for persons with AIDS include: *AIDS in Texas: Facing the Crisis,* an AIDS glossary prepared by the Legislative Task Force on AIDS, Report to the Seventy-first Legislature, January 1989; "Treatment and management of AIDS dementia," prepared by A. Boccellari, Ph.D., Department of Psychiatry, San Francisco, Calif.; "Diagnosis and Management of HIV Primary Dementia," prepared by Francisco Fernandez, MD, St. Luke's Episcopal Hospital, 6720 Bertner, Rm. B-450, Houston, Texas, telephone (713) 791-2665; and an article entitled "Malignant neoplasia in AIDS" by Dennis A. Lowenthal MD and others, in *Infections in Medicine,* April 1987. Other useful resources are *And the Band Played On* by Randy Shilts (Penguin Books, 1988) and *On Borrowed Time: An AIDS Memoir* by Paul Monette (Harcourt Brace Jovanovich, 1988).

CHILDREN OF CANCER PATIENTS: ISSUES AND INTERVENTIONS

Joan Hermann, MSW, ACSW

INTRODUCTION

Social work intervention with the families of young and adolescent children is one of the most exciting areas of oncology social work. Children facing a serious or life-threatening parental illness are considered to be at high risk for adjustment reactions during a cancer experience, and for many years afterwards if the parent should die. Intervention with this group of families represents an opportunity for preventative work that is well within the social work practitioner's repertoire of skills.

For social workers new to the field, it can also create significant anxiety as professionals learn to feel competent with this population. This anxiety is related to three issues. One is an almost primitive fantasy that children can be protected from such a devastating reality as the potential loss of a parent. Unfortunately, this is not possible, but children do possess the capacity to learn to deal with this threat to their daily lives and to their futures. A second source of anxiety is a perceived lack of knowledge and/or skills in working with children. Social workers without direct experience with children may fear that they might unwittingly damage a child if their intervention is incorrect. Fortunately, children are not that fragile and they do not suffer permanent damage because of an ill-conceived explanation or use of language. The third source of anxiety centers on parental resistance to intervention. Most often this is based on anxiety and uncertainty rather than unwillingness to deal with the issue. The task confronting the social worker is to enable parents, as the child's best source of security, to help their child cope. A child's adjustment to catastrophic illness is intimately connected to the quality of parental coping. The area of parental coping is where most social work intervention on behalf of children will occur.

This chapter offers social workers new to oncology basic knowledge upon which to develop intervention skills applicable to this population of vulnerable children and their families. The material is discussed in relation to the predictable phases of the cancer experience: diagnosis, cure, progressive and terminal illness, and bereavement.

ISSUES AT DIAGNOSIS

Giving correct information about the diagnosis of cancer and how it will be treated is the most important step in guiding a child's adjustment. For many parents, this is an extremely difficult task to master as it threatens them at their most vulnerable point. Parents can become overwhelmed, as they incorrectly assume the imagined reactions of their children to be identical to theirs. Social workers need to reassure parents that young children do not have the same intellectual awareness of or emotional reaction to cancer as do adults. For this reason, children usually will not demonstrate the shock, anxiety, and fear of death characteristic of the diagnostic phase. Parents often think that they may be able to shield their child from knowledge of the diagnosis as long as they can continue to behave normally. This is not possible, as life is far from normal for a family grappling with a cancer diagnosis. Children absorb the unspoken anxiety of their parents and intuitively know that something is very wrong. The energy used in trying to keep cancer a secret is an enormous strain. At a minimum, children should be told the name of the disease (cancer), the site (part of the body affected), and how the disease will be treated. The child's most immediate psychological need is for security, so the uncertainties in the child's world need responses. The child's concerns such as "Who will cook dinner if mom's in the hospital?" or "Who will take me to baseball practice?" must be addressed. The child must be given the message that even though the family is faced with a serious problem, parents are still in charge and are planning for the disruption in family life associated with the initial treatment course.

During this period, it is useful to assign children specific, age-appropriate tasks to accommodate the necessary changes in household routines. This helps the child feel included in the family's experience. Adolescents may take on more responsibilities than younger children as is age appropriate. Teenagers should be helped to know that parents are not abdicating their responsibilities, only postponing them for a period of time.

Because of their egocentricity, children also need to be told that it is not anyone's fault that cancer has happened. As in divorce situations, children often think they are the cause of family problems but rarely will ask directly. Children need to know that it is extremely unlikely that the other parent will get sick, and that they themselves will not get cancer. At this stage, a child rarely asks if the parent will die. If the question is asked, parents need to respond with something with which they are comfortable. A social worker may help parents rehearse their answer to this question so that the parents feel prepared and in control. Possible answers might be, "Many people are cured of cancer these days, that's why I'm getting treatment" or "We are all going to die one day. I'll tell you if that is something you should be worrying about."

While questions about death are extremely threatening, parents will feel more in control of themselves and their lives if they are able to deal with their children's questions and fears. Since the primary task of parenthood is to help children cope with life, parents and their children will experience relief in tackling problems together with the implicit message being, "As a family we can cope with this."

Honest communication between parent and child will serve families well throughout the illness experience. Obviously, the explanation of cancer will differ, depending on the child's age and developmental stage. For young children, cancer can be explained as a tumor made up of cells that don't work right and eventually hurt other parts of the body. Older children may need more information; they are exposed to cancer via the lay press, health education in the schools, hearing about others with cancer, or perhaps the experience of cancer in a grandparent or other relative. The principle of giving children appropriate information is sound regardless of prognosis. The focus should be on living with a chronic illness, unless treatment is known to have failed and the focus must shift to dealing with progressive disease and palliation. Social workers can be extremely useful in helping parents to sort out overwhelming feelings and to find appropriate ways to communicate with their children.

It is important for a child to understand how cancer is to be treated and what side effects the parent is likely to experience. Surgery can be explained as an operation in which the doctor removes the tumor; the parent will not be awake so it will not hurt. Because the idea of a parent being "cut open" can produce powerful fantasies in a child, it is important that children be permitted to visit in the hospital as soon after surgery as possible. They should be prepared to see the parent with bandages, I.V. bottles, and so forth. The trappings of hospital care are often fascinating to children, not horrifying as some adults expect. As long as a parent is able to communicate with a child, a hospital visit offers powerful reassurance that the child has not been abandoned.

The side effects of chemotherapy should be explained before they occur so that children know what to expect. Hair loss and nausea can be explained as temporary and a sign that the drugs are working. Children should know that their parent under treatment may be "grouchy" or have less patience and that it is not the child's fault if the parent is more irritable. If radiation therapy is planned, children can be told that side effects will vary, depending on the area of the body being treated. Depending on their age, children should be told that the parent is not "radioactive." It is extremely useful for children to visit the outpatient setting on a day when treatment is not planned. Children should meet the treatment staff (e.g., chemotherapy nurses, radiation therapy technologists), see where the treatment will take place, and be reassured that what is to happen is in the parent's best interest.

A child's ability to master the impact of parental illness will be greatly enhanced by preserving the child's routine as much as possible. Extended family and friends can be called upon to enable the child to continue extracurricular activities, lessons, and so forth so that life remains as much the same as is possible. Young children should not be removed from the family environment, if at all possible. It may be tempting to suggest a visit to a grandparent if a parent is having difficulty with the demands of parenting, but this often reinforces the child's fantasies of abandonment. School-age and adolescent children should continue their studies, with the message that parents expect the same behavior and attention to lessons as before. Social workers can suggest that a parent communicate with the child's teacher or guidance counselor so that they may be alert to a child who is having difficulty at school.

Likewise, parents should adhere to the same guidelines on discipline and other issues as before the illness. This may impose more stress on the well parent, but children will feel out of control if suddenly the same rules no longer apply. Social workers can be helpful during this time by helping parents establish priorities, reach out to extended families (especially for single parents), suggest "family meetings" in which parents and children can discuss issues, and offer support during this very stressful time. Community agencies may be useful for homemaking assistance, help with transportation, and/or other services. Adolescents may feel especially burdened during periods of active treatment because they realistically can assume many parental duties. Although parents can expect more of adolescents, they should be aware that the teenager needs relief from family responsibilities, special "thank you's," and time to be with peers and carry on usual activities. A social worker working with several families may offer group meetings for teens as a means of reducing the isolation that teenagers may be feeling. Social workers can be very helpful in enabling families to make family life accommodations to serious illness. The social work role is one of anticipation and education; parents usually know their children best, but they cannot know the potential effects of serious illness until it is experienced.

A child's developmental needs continue in spite of parental illness, so social workers need to be aware of some general principles. Helping seriously ill parents support their children's developmental needs can be challenging but ultimately reassuring to parents struggling to cope. The way a child reacts is most often reflected in his or her behavior. Young children may appear to lose ground if their world is threatened. For instance, children who are fully toilet trained may start having accidents. Two- and 3-year-olds, who normally are very adventuresome in exploring their environments, may become unusually clingy. First-graders who have adjusted well to starting school may resist going to school and display exaggerated separation anxiety. For children who cannot articulate their worries, these behaviors clue parents to anxieties about changes in the household or in their relationship to their parents. During these times, parents may need to offer extra attention to their children. If a parent is feeling too ill, other family members may be called upon to temporarily help manage.

School-age children have the advantage of being able to verbalize their feelings and also have more resources outside of their immediate families to help them cope. School personnel should be informed of parental illness so the child's responses can be understood within that context.

Parental illness can be particularly difficult for adolescents, who are in a developmental stage of separation from parental figures. It is typical for teenagers to test parental limits and to gradually achieve more self-confidence in their desire for independence. When this process is interrupted by illness, teenagers can experience ambivalence and resentment, especially if they are called upon to take over parental responsibilities. Social workers, by helping parents anticipate the developmental needs of their children in relation to chronic illness, can make a substantial difference in how parents encourage that process.

ISSUES OF SURVIVORSHIP

Nearly 50% of cancer patients treated today will achieve long-term survival or cure, so it is important to consider the impact of this on developing children. For the parent, believing that the disease is under control or cured is often difficult. Many people describe the pervasive anxiety that characterizes medical follow-up appointments. Fortunately, most children react to what they experience and if a parent looks and feels well, the child often ceases to feel threatened. There are situations, however, in which children can have difficulty. Depending on age, some children may have made significant gains in assuming more responsibilities and feel resentful if the parent is not able to appreciate their growing independence. Children can also experience anger toward the well parent, as it is now psychologically safe to express such feelings. If a parent has been idealized during illness, children can feel tremendously guilty about angry feelings and need permission to have such negative thoughts. No family is ever the same following a cancer diagnosis, so children will have had to adjust to whatever changes were necessary in family routines and roles. Children who assumed responsibilities of the sick parent can develop a pseudo-maturity that is inappropriate to the parents' recovery. This situation needs monitoring in order to prevent "parentification" of the child. The impact of extended long-term treatment may have financial and social implications. A troubled marital relationship may worsen or dissolve and children may have to endure that threat to their identities and security.

Because of the nature of thc health care delivery system, social workers are less frequently consulted about the problems associated with cancer survivorship. Social work departments in hospitals need to consider what the absence of such services will mean to children and their families. Other models of intervention might be considered if staffing does not permit reaching out to cancer survivors. An example is educational materials that are automatically distributed and available in the oncologist's office. Integrating content concerning children into support/educational groups and dialogue with educators and school counselors are other examples of interventions that can be useful to families struggling to deal with the long-term implications of cancer diagnosis and treatment.

ISSUES OF PROGRESSIVE ILLNESS

The ability of a social worker to be truly helpful to families facing progressive disease will depend on many factors, not the least of which is the social worker's ability to connect with a family in crisis. Families are often more amenable to help during crisis points and social workers should take advantage of this in assessing needs of children. Even if children have been told very little about the parent's condition, they often know a great deal based on the parent's appearance, behavior, and interaction with medical caregivers. The social worker's role at this point in the illness is an enabling and educational one. Parents need suggestions as to how they will facilitate the child's coping. Social workers are sometimes uncomfortable with such an active role, fearing that the clients' right to self-determination will be displaced. However, it is important for social workers to realize that parents have no way of knowing about how children best cope with this experience. It is the social worker's responsibility to share information about how other families have coped, so parents can make an informed choice about how to best help their children.

Children should be given information gradually, and it should be tailored to the reality of the medical situation. For instance, if a parent has experienced a first recurrence of the disease and will require more aggressive treatment, children can be told that the doctors will be using "stronger medicines" to control the situation. If a parent has widely metastatic disease, children can be told that the doctors are worried that the medicines are not working as well as they did in the past. Children most often take their cues from what they physically experience. If a parent looks well, as some people with advanced disease do, a child may not realize the meaning of disease progression. In such situations, it is even more important that communication continue to occur. It is always useful to solicit a child's perception of what is happening with a sick parent so that information can then be tailored to that reality rather than something which the child has not even considered. For example, a simple "What have you thought about how Mom is doing?" can be the starting point in the dialogue.

In contrast to other illnesses, cancer usually occurs over a prolonged period of time. Children and adults will have a period of time in which to prepare for the loss. For a child, the loss begins when the parent is no longer able to interact with the child in the usual way. If Dad is too sick to go to a ball game, an uncle might substitute. Mom may not be able to shop for a prom dress, so another relative may offer to do so. While it is healthy for a child to be able to adapt to these parental substitutions, they engender feelings that must be acknowledged. The well parent might say, "It is great that Uncle Harry likes baseball too, but I know you would rather be going with your Dad. It makes me angry too that he is so sick." Children need permission to be angry. While it is not a "rational" response to be angry at someone who is ill, it is nevertheless a very common and human response. Children who are unable to express these feelings bear a far greater burden and the potential for psychological damage is more likely.

A child can begin to withdraw from parental relationships, especially if a parent is unable to physically respond to a child's needs. At this point, it can be useful to give the child certain tasks that he or she can do with the sick parent. This enables the child to stay connected to his or her parent, albeit in a different manner, and it supports the child's mourning process with positive memories of the relationship.

ISSUES OF TERMINAL ILLNESS AND BEREAVEMENT

A child must be prepared for the expected death of a parent. This preparation will be much easier if the child has been included in the illness experience from the beginning. If this has not been the case, parents usually realize at this point that children must be addressed. It is atypical for the sick parent to be capable of direct interaction with the child about his or her own death. For parents who feel guilty about their inability to take on this very difficult task, the social worker may suggest that they write letters to their children expressing their love and hopes for them. Some parents make video tapes for their children. These kinds of activities can do much to help children retain a positive memory of a parent they have lost.

The well parent or another relative may be faced with telling the child about an impending death. Obviously, this is a source of tremendous anxiety. If possible, parents should be encouraged to do this themselves, as they will achieve a tremendous sense of mastery by doing so. A parent may need a social worker's help to prepare for the conversation, but the social worker should not attempt to take over this responsibility unless the parent is totally unable to do so. The social worker may help the parent to role play how the dialogue may go, so the parent feels as prepared as possible. Depending on age, the course of the illness, and family circumstances, a child may have already begun the process of withdrawal from the sick parent. If this has happened, it is useful to use that reality in the service of the child's understanding. For example, saying "You know that Daddy has not been able to play baseball with you for a while" may help reinforce the child's understanding of what will happen.

The reactions of children to impending parental death depend on several factors: age, how much preparation they have received since the initial diagnosis, their relationships to both the sick and well parents, their own coping mechanisms, and the availability of social support. Some important concepts for parents to know include the following:

- Prior to age 5 or 6, children are unable to comprehend the finality and universality of death. Children will often ask when "Mommy is coming back."
- Death can be explained as not being able to see, hear, feel, be with us anymore. For example, "We will not see Mommy anymore, but we will be able to remember her through pictures and stories."
- Illness and death are not anyone's fault. "We did not cause Dad to be sick (or die) when we were angry with him" and "It is okay to be angry that Dad died. He loved you very much and did not want to leave" may be appropriate responses.

Social workers can be enormously helpful to parents facing this situation. The most pressing need is to give information in anticipation of family bereavement rituals. The issue of a child's attendance at the parent's funeral is a useful example, as this is typically controversial. This is an area, however, where social workers can share their knowledge about children's reactions to funerals, so that parents can make a decision that is right for them. While children need preparation for a funeral, they tend to receive considerable benefit from attendance. Funerals can be explained as "The way we say goodbye to someone we love." It can be useful to explain about who will be there, what the service will be like, that people will be upset, and how the child is expected to act. The younger a child is, the harder it will be to understand death. A funeral is a tremendous help in the child's reality testing of that event. When the 5-year-old cannot understand that Mommy will not be there for Christmas, the memory of the funeral can be reinforced as a way to help the young child understand. Although parents may be tempted to exclude children from the funeral ritual, feeling that it may be too emotional, confusing, or upsetting, it should be pointed out that children may interpret this to mean that death is so dreadful that it is not possible to cope with it or certainly for them to be able to deal with it. Parents may also unwittingly give the message that the child is not part of the family and that their relationship to the deceased is unimportant. Families will do what they can tolerate, but the exclusion of children from this significant event can have lasting, long-term repercussions.

Obviously, death will be explained to children according to a family's cultural and religious beliefs. For families with a strong spiritual life, the combination of death with afterlife is a more comforting association than for families for whom such an idea is less certain or unacceptable. For those families, children are better able to tolerate an honest "I don't know" than explanations that do not fit into a family's belief system. The social worker's belief system is immaterial, but it can be useful to point out some of the areas of conflict that some religious beliefs can produce for children. Examples are "God chose Mommy to be with Him in Heaven" (resulting in anger at God) or "Daddy is watching you from Heaven" (which can interfere with spontaneity and the natural experimentation of childhood).

Children are often quite sensitive to incongruities in the way adults deal with death. They wonder about the family gathering that often occurs following the burial, as this event can look to them like a party. Likewise, adults may misunderstand the grief of a child and incorrectly assume that it will follow the same pattern as that of an adult. Children express their grief in abbreviated doses and are incapable of the intensity of expression characteristic of adults. For instance, children will cry for brief periods of time but will typically use the safety of play activity to manage their feelings. Children's sadness and grief will be manifested in their behavior, which can become regressed or provocative as a way of signaling their distress. Parents know their children best, but it is useful to help a parent put their child's behavior into the perspective of what is usual in understanding how to best respond. Parents should be reminded to model their own feelings for their children, as by saying "I feel so sad today that Mom isn't with us anymore," especially if a child is not sharing his or her feelings with anyone. The surviving parent should remember to tell the children that death is no one's fault, and that specifically the children did not cause Mom or Dad to die. This is an irrational thought, but it is one of the most common observed in children dealing with the death of a parent. Social workers can do much to help parents prepare for this uncharted territory so that they are as helpful to their children as possible.

Parents also need to be educated about the typical course for childhood mourning. Children often seem to have a more protracted grief experience than do adults due to developmental changes and the child's changing ability to understand and process the death as they mature. Children can experience feelings of intense grief during periods of their lives in which the parent would have participated, such as a graduation, holidays, or the anniversary of the death.

Social workers also need to realize that surviving parents will be unable to facilitate the children's mourning process if their own bereavement needs are unmet. A parent who has no outlet for feelings will be unable to respond to the needs of his or her children. The social worker who is offering bereavement services facilitates a resolution for the entire family.

INTERVENTIONS

Many interventions are available to social workers involved in the management of serious loss for children. These include educational materials, individual and family counseling, support groups, and the use of the hospital environment to reinforce reality. The nature of those services will depend on the nature of the contract between client and social worker. Many families will take advantage of social workers' help, but some families will resist all efforts. While this is frustrating, parents generally do the best they can; social workers who are too aggressive in their desire to help will usually get a negative response. Families may isolate themselves and a relationship that might be less threatening after a death has occurred is thwarted. Families who are resistant to intervention during the illness might accept reading materials and be responsive to a social workers' outreach following a death. Hospice programs offer routine bereavement follow-up. Social work follow-up can be extremely useful for non-hospice families.

Support groups are extremely helpful in all stages of the cancer experience, but especially so with the bereaved. While social workers can do a great deal by way of education about what to expect, there is nothing quite like that information coming from someone who has experienced it. The person who believes that his or her loss will never be resolved can discover that many different kinds of resolution are possible. Bereavement groups are also quite helpful for children. For young children, they typically take the form of play or art therapy and offer the bereaved child an acceptable way to move through the feelings of aloneness and abandonment that the loss of a parent produces. Information about such groups can be obtained by contacting the social work departments of major cancer centers, hospice programs, the National Association of Oncology Social Workers, and the American Cancer Society.

In addition to such traditional services, social workers can be helpful in utilizing the available medical environment to help children understand. Family meetings with the physician can be arranged so that children have an opportunity to learn what to expect. Hospital visits to sick parents can be arranged without fear of damage to children. As long as a parent is able to communicate, such visits are extremely useful to the child and reinforce reality in a very concrete way. If a parent is not conscious, a visit can still be a powerful way for a child to test reality, as long as the child is prepared for what to expect.

CONCLUSION

Social workers should know that only in recent years have the needs of children of adult patients been recognized. Much remains to be learned, especially in the area of research designed to demonstrate the effectiveness of intervention with this group of children. What is known from clinical experience is that social workers have the opportunity to positively influence the quality of the families' experience with catastrophic illness. In dealing with the impact of cancer, social workers usually have the advantage of a process that occurs over time. During that experience, with its predictable crisis points, parents can be helped to monitor and engage their children in ways of coping with the potential of serious loss. Families bring their own internal resources to the experience. Within the context of a supportive relationship, they can often begin to utilize these strengths in helping children understand the reality of serious illness. Social workers can sometimes feel immobilized by the challenges faced by these young families and the ultimate unfairness of life. However, it is in helping families meet the challenges that the unfairness becomes tolerable and the impact of cancer is reduced to problems that are amenable to solutions. The loss of a parent in childhood is a devastating reality, but social workers have much to offer in helping families confront the tasks of illness and move toward healing and resolution.

SUGGESTED READINGS

RESOURCES FOR PROFESSIONALS

American Cancer Society. *Cancer Facts and Figures.* Atlanta, Ga: American Cancer Society; 1992.

Baker J, Sedney MA, Gross E. Psychological tasks for bereaved children. *Am J Orthopsychiatry.* 1992;62:105-116.

Bowlby J. *Attachment and Loss.* vols I–III. New York, NY: Basic Books; 1980.

Furman E. *A Child's Parent Dies: Studies in Childhood Bereavement.* New Haven, Conn: Yale University Press; 1974.

Johnson P, Rosenblatt P. Grief following childhood loss of a parent. *Psychotherapy.* 1981; 35:419-425.

Lonetto R. *Children's Conceptions of Death.* New York, NY: Springer Publishing Company; 1980.

Osterweis M, Soloman F, Green M, eds. *Bereavement: Reactions, Consequences, and Care.* Washington, DC: National Academy Press; 1984.

Raphael B. Young child and the death of a parent. In: *The Place of Attachment and Human Behavior.* New York, NY: Basic Books; 1982.

Silverman P, Worden J. Children's reactions in the early months after the death of a parent. *Am J Orthopsychiatry.* 1992;62:93-104.

Simos B. *A Time to Grieve.* New York, NY: Family Service Association

of America; 1979.
Tessman L. *Children of Parting Parents.* New York and London: Jason Aronson; 1968.
Wass H, Coor C, eds. *Childhood and Death.* Washington, DC: Hemisphere Publishing Corp; 1984.
Wass H, Coor C, eds. *Helping Children Cope with Death: Guidelines and Resources.* Washington, DC: Hemisphere Publishing Corp; 1984.
Worden J. *Grief Counseling and Grief Therapy.* New York, NY: Springer Publishing Company; 1982.

RESOURCES FOR PARENTS AND CHILDREN

Bernstein J. *Loss and How to Cope with It.* Boston, Mass: Houghton Mifflin; 1977.
Coburn J. *Anne and the Sand Dobbies.* New York, NY: Seabury Press; 1964.
Grollman E. *Talking About Death: A Dialogue Between Parent and Child.* Boston, Mass: Beacon Press; 1976.
Krementz J. *How It Feels When a Parent Dies.* New York, NY: MacMillan Publishing Co; 1976.
LeShan E. *Learning to Say Goodbye: When a Parent Dies.* New York, NY: MacMillan Publishing Co; 1976.
LeShan E. *When a Parent Is Very Sick.* Boston, Mass: Little, Brown and Co; 1986.
Stein S. *About Dying: An Open Family Book for Parents.* New York, NY: Walker and Co; 1974.
Viorst J. *The Tenth Good Thing About Barnie.* New York, NY: Atheneum; 1971.

PROGRAMS FOR ADULTS WITH CANCER

Catherine S. Cordoba, MSW, ACSW

People have formed various associations that have a number of programs and services to assist those facing cancer with their adjustment to the illness and to ease their sense of aloneness. In this section, the role of voluntary organizations will be reviewed along with the functions of groups, home health agencies, and hospices.

VOLUNTARY ORGANIZATIONS IN ONCOLOGY

Voluntary organizations generally offer individuals direct opportunities to help shape services and to provide one-to-one service to other people. They have been defined as nongovernmental, nonprofit social service organizations that seek to assist others directly or indirectly. These agencies have always been central to social work.[1]

Many voluntary organizations have been formed in the health field, particularly in the area of cancer where they fulfill an important role. With the growth of the consumer movement, increasing restrictions in health care services, and with a lack of response to many of the needs of persons facing cancer, more and more have been created.

The American Cancer Society is one of the oldest and largest voluntary health agencies in the United States. It was organized in 1913 by a group of physicians and lay persons and today is a national society with 57 chartered divisions (usually grouped by state) and more than 3 300 units or local offices.

The Society's purpose is to control cancer by carrying out programs of research, education (both for the public and for professionals), and services for cancer patients and their families. Thousands of volunteers are involved in implementing these programs. Some of the special programs to meet concrete needs and address psychosocial issues include information and referral services (Resources, Information and Guidance or RIG), transportation to and from treatment, supportive services for those facing breast cancer (Reach to Recovery), other patient-to-patient visitor programs such as Cansurmount or CanSupport, patient and family education materials, courses on cancer (I Can Cope), and programs on appearance (Look Good, Feel Better).

Other voluntary agencies specifically addressing the needs of cancer patients include: the Leukemia Society of America, Candlelighters Foundation, the United Ostomy Association, the International Association of Laryngectomies, and the National Coalition for Cancer Survivorship. Cancer Care, Make Today Count, Corporate Angel Network, the YWCA's Encore program, and many other associations at local and state levels are also involved in assisting cancer patients and their families. All these organizations sponsor a variety of activities ranging from practical assistance and supportive services to advocacy to influence government policies. (See Resources in Cancer Care for Adults and Children for more information on these organizations.)

INVOLVEMENT FOR SOCIAL WORKERS

It is important that oncology social workers become involved with organizations concerned with cancer in order to lend their expertise and knowledge to help in the development of programs and services. By volunteering, they can advance a better understanding of the psychosocial impact of cancer and bring in standards of social work. Social workers can strengthen the role of other volunteers by contributing their "science" of helping. They can provide organization and direction to charitable impulses.

Most voluntary organizations face a continual problem of how to involve those in lower socioeconomic groups. While there is no substitute for the real thing, social workers can serve as advocates for the poor, the underserved, and the disenfranchised; they also can provide assistance in involving these important constituents.

Service committees of local units of the American Cancer Society are particularly in need of the participation of social workers. By becoming involved as volunteers, social workers can facilitate the creation of services to meet needs and can encourage broad interpretation of policies and procedures that will aid the expansion of services to patients and families. By maintaining focus on patient needs, they can help avoid concentration on process rather than results.

Social workers can offer consultation and support to staff persons who may have little background and experience in working with patients. They can assist with volunteer training, support groups, educational forums, and provide individual counseling or back-up on difficult cases.

In addition to working in a direct service area, social workers need to expand their spheres of influence and become involved in policy areas, that is, in the inner workings of these associations where the decisions are made. Often this means they need to involve themselves in areas such as organization and structure, recruitment of volunteers, fund-raising, public relations, strategic planning, legislation, etc. The skills that social workers have, especially those of facilitation and negotiation, can be used to advantage in many areas and can help cancer-concerned organizations run more smoothly and become more effective.

GROUPS

One response to the turmoil following a cancer diagnosis has been the formation of various kinds of support groups. These groups are sponsored not only by voluntary organizations, but also by acute care hospitals and community-based health care organizations. Groups can be categorized generally into three basic types:

1. Self-help or mutual support groups made up of patients and/or family members who share a common situation or condition
2. Counseling/therapy groups that are usually led by social workers in hospital settings but also involve psychologists, other types of counselors, and nurses
3. Education/discussion groups involving a variety of professionals and lay persons.[2]

Cancer support groups provide a place where cancer patients can talk with others who are having the same experiences. Mutual support can lessen the stress of a common predicament as people facing similar problems can often be a resource for one another. Group members can provide each other with ideas, facts, beliefs, and resources that they have found helpful in coping with similar problems. By listening to others discuss feelings they may have deemed inappropriate, members often get more in touch with their own feelings.[3]

Groups offer a safe, supportive atmosphere where persons affected by cancer can discuss difficult decisions they need to make and life changes they are undergoing. They can also help participants learn about themselves in relation to cancer. Another advantage to the group experience is that it can increase social activity at a time when former activities often slow down because of the illness.[2]

Self-help groups are organized by and composed of members who share the work and responsibility for the group; the expertise and problem-solving stem from the members' experiences. These groups foster a sense of belonging that is especially important to persons facing cancer. While professionals rarely provide leadership to these groups, many self-help groups have been started by health professionals. Health professionals often serve as advisors or facilitators.[4] Oncology social workers can be particularly helpful to such groups by providing consultation on group leadership, possible themes and topics for discussion, suggestions for handling difficult members and dysfunctional actions, ways to curb absences and dropouts, and how to find available resources.

Professionally led cancer support groups and counseling groups differ from traditional psychotherapy groups that are formed for persons experiencing mental health problems or problems in relationships. The function of a psychotherapy group is to foster interpersonal learning so that its members can grow and change. Although participants in cancer support groups may also have mental health problems, generally they do not come to a group to deal with these problems; they come to deal with cancer.

People facing cancer usually have a great need for information, and groups that focus on providing information can be extremely helpful to both patients and their families. Participants can learn about the disease, treatment options, and resources. They can learn to more effectively deal with the health care system. Education and discussion groups can provide a nonthreatening environment where patients can ask health professionals not involved in their care questions they might be reluctant to ask their own physicians. Some patients do not know what questions to ask and need more information before they can do so. In groups set up to provide information in a supportive atmosphere, patients can clear up misconceptions, learn effective ways of coping, and gain a greater sense of mastery over their illness. Family members can gain a better understanding of what the patient is experiencing, learn about ways of caring for the patient, and become better equipped to offer assistance. The American Cancer Society, the National Cancer Institute, and other cancer organizations have free, informative materials that can supplement content in these groups.

HOME HEALTH AGENCIES

Home care may be thought of as "hospitals without walls," or "the extension of the hospital into the community."[5] Home care programs are not new. The earliest one in the United States appears to have been established in 1796 at the Boston Dispensary.[6] In recent years, virtually all serious illnesses have been handled in hospitals because of their concentration of medical services. However, cancer increasingly is being treated on an outpatient basis and patients are being discharged from inpatient care earlier due to fiscal constraints. Many cancer patients are left with no alternatives but home care.

Psychologically, patients usually fare better at home and have more control over what happens to them. There are some disadvantages, however. Family routines can be seriously disrupted and care of the patient can become a burden for the family, especially when caretakers are elderly. Some patients do not have anyone to assist them at home.

TRANSITION FROM HOSPITAL TO HOME

The transition from hospital to home requires a coordinated plan of care geared to individual needs. A social work assessment is a crucial part of the plan. Many families have concerns about their ability to care for patients and to meet their needs. Family members may be unprepared for changes in their pattern of living. The patient may be wary of leaving the hospital. These and other concerns expressed by patients and families need to be discussed. The family needs to know what to expect once the patient is home.

It can be helpful for a social worker to review a daily routine with the family and eliminate obstacles before the patient leaves the hospital. Often, the caretaker works outside the home and may be fearful of leaving the patient alone or may feel overwhelmed by all that has to be done.

Helping caretakers find other resources such as friends, relatives, neighbors, and church and fraternal organizations can help a great deal. The American Cancer Society offers free booklets on caring for patients at home that can be extremely helpful to caretakers.

The hospital, the home health agency, the family, and the patient have to be involved in joint planning. Arrangements for needed services not provided by the home health agency such as homemakers, transportation, meals, and special equipment or supplies, should be made before discharge from the hospital. However, this assumes the patient has a family or someone to provide care at home. Planning for the person who lives alone requires a great deal of forethought and ingenuity.

To ensure continuity of care, the information provided in referral to a home health agency must be comprehensive as to the type of personnel and services needed and medications, including potential side effects. All home health personnel need to know what patients have been told about their condition and treatment procedures. It is equally important to know the patients' and families' reactions to this information. Home health personnel can be much more effective when they are given as much background information as possible.[7] Developing a total home care plan before the patient is discharged is critical to the success of post-hospital treatment. The social work assessment is vital to the plan.

TYPES OF HOME HEALTH AGENCIES

There are four general types of home care providers:

- Public agencies operated by state or local units such as health and welfare departments
- Nonprofit nongovernmental agencies such as Visiting Nurse Associations (VNA) or agencies located in hospitals, skilled nursing facilities or rehabilitation facilities, and private nonprofit agencies operated by individuals
- Proprietary agencies including all privately owned profit making agencies
- Combined agencies operated by an organization with dual sponsorship by a governmental agency and a voluntary agency, such as a health department and a VNA.[8]

SERVICES PROVIDED IN HOME HEALTH CARE

Home health care agencies are state licensed to provide many in-home services including skilled nursing care, home health aides, homemaker services, physical and occupational therapy, social work services, and nutritional counseling. Services, which must be authorized by the patient's physician, are financed through private insurance, Medicare, Medicaid, patient fees, and donations. Visiting Nurse Associations are nonprofit home health agencies that are supported by United Way and the other funding methods previously listed.

Not all services provided by home health agencies are reimbursable and, as a result, the number and kinds of services vary considerably. Nursing personnel are generally permanent members of a home health agency staff but occupational, physical, and speech therapists and social workers may be employed in other agencies or be in private practice. These professionals may provide services on a contractual basis or on a fee-for-service basis.[8]

COST REIMBURSEMENT

Although the cost of care can be reduced by treating the patient in the home, reimbursement mechanisms to pay for home care have yet to be resolved. Private insurance companies, as a rule, do not pay for home care although skilled nursing care is provided under some plans. Some patients, desperate for any kind of assistance in the home, use their insurance benefit to hire a skilled nurse when they may only need the service of a homemaker or home health aide. This is a costly alternative that can strain the limits of a patient's insurance coverage.

Medicare can pay for home health visits if all these conditions are met:

- The patient is confined to the home and needs intermittent skilled nursing care, physical therapy, or speech therapy
- A physician determines the patient needs home health care and sets up a home care plan
- The home health agency providing the care is participating in Medicare.

If a patient needs any of the above services, Medicare may also pay for occupational therapy, etc.

Medicare home health services do not include coverage for general household services, meal preparation, shopping, or other home care services furnished mainly to assist people in meeting personal or family needs. Other home health services not covered by Medicare include 24-hour-a-day nursing care at home, drugs and biologicals, meals delivered to the home, and blood transfusions.[9] Specific information about Medicare coverage can be obtained from any Social Security Administration Office.

Many cancer patients who are confined to their homes and who need care do not qualify under Medicare because they are deemed to need custodial care, not skilled nursing care. Patients in hospice programs certified by Medicare, however, can be provided with "appropriate custodial care."[9] The lack of reimbursement for home care services poses particular problems for the chronically ill. Many may need only minimal assistance, such as with personal care, cleaning, meal preparation, and shopping, in order to remain in their homes with some comfort and dignity. Other resources in the community should be explored including Medicaid, organizations serving cancer patients, churches, social agencies, and fraternal groups.

Quality of Home Care

In summary, the quality of home care and the quality of life can best be achieved through:

- Comprehensive planning
- Counseling and preparation of the patient, family, and the personnel in contact with them
- A good communication system for the provider of care
- Coordination of all aspects of care.[7]

HOSPICES

Hospice has been defined as a concept, not a place. Hospices emphasize palliative and supportive care to meet the special needs of patients and their families during the final stages of an illness.[10] The primary goals of hospices are to control pain, ensure general spiritual and mental comfort, assure a dignified death for the patient, and give support and comfort to the family.

The hospice movement began as an effort to improve the care of dying patients. As a result, a major focus of hospice care has been the emotional effects of the illness on the dying patient and the family.[11] Hospices today are professional, well-organized resources for the terminally ill.

CARDINAL PRINCIPLES OF HOSPICE

Cardinal principles of hospice care have been delineated as:

- The scope of hospice care is terminal illness; care is directed primarily at palliation.
- A key feature of care is that it is directed primarily at symptom control. Symptoms are considered to include psychosocial problems as well as physical complaints.
- Hospice service must be provided at varying levels of care in multiple settings (inpatient and outpatient) and must be available 24 hours a day.
- The patient and the family are the unit of care.
- There must be a multidisciplinary team approach.[12]

HOSPICE COSTS COVERED BY MEDICARE

Hospice care includes home care, inpatient care, and a variety of services not otherwise covered under Medicare. Medicare hospital insurance helps pay for hospice care if all of three conditions are met:

- A doctor certifies that a patient is terminally ill
- A patient chooses to receive care from a hospice instead of standard Medicare benefits for the terminal illness
- Care is provided by a Medicare-participating hospice program.[8]

The following are covered under Medicare as part of hospice care:

- Nursing and doctors' services
- Drugs, medical supplies, and appliances
- Physical therapy, occupational therapy, and speech-language therapy
- Home health aide and homemaker services
- Medical social services and counseling
- Short-term inpatient care, including respite care.

RESOURCES FOR CARE

A list of hospice programs can be obtained from the National Hospice Organization, Suite 307, 1901 North Fort Myer Drive, Arlington, VA 22209. American Cancer Society offices will also be able to provide information about local hospice programs. This information should be added to the social worker's resource files along with the criteria for admission and procedures.

If a hospice program is not available, social workers should explore alternatives. Sometimes patients or families inquiring about hospice care have only fragmentary knowledge of such programs and may be seeking some component of hospice care available through other community resources. The best solution can be found by assessing the situation and working with patients and their families.

CONCLUSION

Cancer is a complex, long-term illness requiring a wide array of programs and services. As care of the cancer patient has moved into the community, the programs offered by voluntary organizations, home health agencies, and hospices assume increasing importance. Social workers must be knowledgeable about the many programs, assist patients and families in accessing them, become involved and, in some instances, advocate for the development of new programs to address existing gaps in service.

REFERENCES

1. Tropman E, Tropman J. Voluntary agencies. In: *Encyclopedia of Social Work, 18th ed, vol 2*. Silver Springs, Md: National Association of Social Workers; 1987: 825-842.

2. Cordoba C, Shear M, Fobair P, Hall J. *Cancer Support Groups: Practice Handbook.* Oakland, Calif: American Cancer Society California Division; 1984.

3. Shulman L, Gitterman A. The life model, mutual aid, and the mediating function. In: Gitterman A, Shulman L, eds. *Mutual Aid Groups and the Life Cycle.* Itasca, Ill: F.E. Peacock Publishers, Inc; 1986.

4. Project of Self-Help Clearing House. San Francisco, Calif: Mental Health Association of San Francisco; 1985.

5. Eichwald H. An organized home care program. In: Prichard E et al., eds. *Home Care: Living With Dying*. New York, NY: Columbia Univer-

sity Press; 1979: 148-152.
6. Hailperin C. 25 years of home care services. In: Prichard E et al., eds. *Home Care: Living With Dying*. New York, NY: Columbia University Press; 1979: 137-147.
7. Clifford I. Comprehensive planning for care and the home health agency. In: Prichard E, et al., eds. *Home Care: Living With Dying*. New York, NY: Columbia University Press; 1979: 223-231.
8. Spiegel A. *Home Healthcare: Home Birthing to Hospice Care*. Owings Mill, Md: National Health Publishing; 1983.
9. *Health Care Financing Administration Medicare Handbook*. Baltimore, Md: US Department of Health and Human Services; 1990.
10. Abdellah F, Harper B, Lunceford J. *Hospice Care in the United States*. Baltimore, Md: Health Care Financing Administration, US Department of Health and Human Services; 1982.
11. Kane R, Klein S, Bernstein L, Rothenberg R, Wales J. Hospice role in alleviating the emotional stress of terminal patients and their families. *Medical Care;* 1985; 23:189-197.
12. Zimmerman J. *Hospice: Complete Care for the Terminally Ill, 2nd ed*. Baltimore, Munich: Urban and Scwarzenberg, Inc; 1986.

THE MEDICAL DIAGNOSIS AND TREATMENT OF CHILDHOOD CANCER

Philip A. Pizzo, MD

OVERVIEW OF PEDIATRIC MALIGNANCIES

Fortunately, the incidence of childhood cancer is uncommon. In the United States, approximately 7800 new cases of cancer were diagnosed in 1992, or fewer than 1% of all malignancies. Nonetheless, a diagnosis of cancer has devastating implications for the child, the family, and the community. During the past decades, major strides in the treatment of children with cancer have been made. In the 1990s, more than 50% of children diagnosed with cancer may be cured. Still, many children diagnosed today face a potentially fatal outcome and nearly all experience side effects of therapy. These side effects can be acute, chronic, extremely incapacitating, and detrimental to growth and development. All persons involved in the care and treatment of children with cancer should be aware of the rationale behind current therapeutic strategies and understand their risks and benefits. While the future might bring ways to lessen toxicity and improve treatment efficacy, the current approaches to therapy, though highly successful, place tremendous demands upon the patient, the family, and the medical team. The insights gained from research and the development of effective therapies for pediatric malignancies have formed the foundation for the principles of pediatric oncology, as well as guideposts for the treatment of adults with cancer.

EPIDEMIOLOGY

The cancers that occur in children differ significantly from those that arise in adults. The most notable difference is the initial response of most childhood cancers to current therapeutic modalities, resulting in a significant number of cures. This encouraging aspect of treatment relates to the nature of the cancers that occur in children. Cancers of epithelial or differentiated cells predominate in adults, and cancers of embryonal or developing cells and tissues predominate in children. Pediatric malignancies are characterized by a high growth fraction or a higher rate of tumor cell multiplication, enabling the tumors to increase in size more quickly than in many adult malignancies. Unlike in adults, pediatric malignancies tend to be generalized or systemic illnesses at the time they are diagnosed. A tumor in a child that appears to be localized to bone or to a soft tissue nearly always involves microscopic spread to other body organs, although this may be undetectable at the time of initial diagnosis.

Age, sex, race, and geography are important factors in defining pediatric malignancies. Table 1 presents the cancers that predominate in children by age and site. Some cancers that are observed soon after birth (e.g., neuroblastoma or retinoblastoma) suggest a genetic basis for their occurrence. Other malignancies appear to peak during early childhood (e.g., acute lymphoblastic leukemia), whereas others tend to arise during the periods of growth and development associated with adolescence (e.g., osteosarcoma, Ewing's sarcoma, and rhabdomyosarcoma). Age can also influence the outcome for the child with a malignancy. For example, children younger than 1 year of age with neuroblastoma tend to fare well, whereas the prognosis is much poorer for children with the same tumor who are older than 2 years of age. The incidence of pediatric malignancies appears to be slightly higher in males, for reasons that are not clear.

Race is also an important factor in childhood cancers. For example, the incidence of cancer in black children is 80% that of the incidence in white children, largely because of lower incidence of acute leukemia, lymphoma, Ewing's sarcoma, and malignant melanoma.

Notable geographic differences in the rate of childhood malignancies have been observed. For example, although retinoblastoma (a tumor of the eye) accounts for only 4% of childhood cancers in the United States, its incidence is far more common in India. Burkitt's lymphoma accounts for nearly half of the childhood cancers in Uganda, but is relatively rare outside of the so-called "Burkitt's Belt" of central Africa. Some of these differences are due to genetic or environmental factors (ecogenetics) that may interact and contribute to the development of a malignancy.

Table 1
PREDOMINANT PEDIATRIC CANCERS BY AGE AND SITE*

TUMORS	NEWBORN (<1 yr)	INFANT (1–3 yr)	CHILDREN (3–11 yr)	ADOLESCENTS & YOUNG ADULTS (12–21 yr)
HEMATOLOGIC MALIGNANCIES				
Leukemias	Congenital leukemia AML AMMoL	ALL AML CML, juvenile	ALL AML	AML ALL
Lymphomas	Very rare	Lymphoblastic	Lymphoblastic Undifferentiated	Lymphoblastic Undifferentiated Burkitt's Hodgkin's disease
SOLID TUMORS				
Central nervous system	Medulloblastoma Ependymoma Astrocytoma Choroid plexus papilloma	Medulloblastoma Ependymoma Astrocytoma Choroid plexus papilloma	Cerebellar astrocytoma Medulloblastoma Astrocytoma Ependymoma Craniopharyngioma	Cerebellar astrocytoma Astrocytoma Craniopharyngioma Medulloblastoma
Head and neck	Retinoblastoma Rhabdomyosarcoma Neuroblastoma MNET	Retinoblastoma Rhabdomyosarcoma Neuroblastoma	Rhabdomyosarcoma Lymphoma	Lymphoma Rhabdomyosarcoma
Thorax	Neuroblastoma Teratoma	Neuroblastoma Teratoma	Lymphoma Neuroblastoma Rhabdomyosarcoma	Lymphoma Ewing's sarcoma Rhabdomyosarcoma
Abdomen	Neuroblastoma Mesoblastic nephroma Hepatoblastoma Wilms' tumor (>6 mos)	Neuroblastoma Wilms' tumor Hepatoblastoma Leukemia†	Neuroblastoma Wilms' tumor Lymphoma Hepatoma	Lymphoma Hepatocellular carcinoma Rhabdomyosarcoma
Gonads	Yolk sac tumor of testis (endodermal sinus tumor) Teratoma Sarcoma Botryoids Neuroblastoma	Rhabdomyosarcoma Yolk sac tumor of testis Clear cell sarcoma of kidney	Rhabdomyosarcoma	Rhabdomyosarcoma Dysgerminoma Teratocarcinoma, teratoma Embryonal carcinoma of testis Embryonal cell and endodermal sinus tumors of ovary
Extremities	Fibrosarcoma	Fibrosarcoma Rhabdomyosarcoma	Rhabdomyosarcoma Ewing's sarcoma	Osteosarcoma Rhabdomyosarcoma Ewing's sarcoma

* From: Pizzo PA, Horowitz ME, Poplack DG, Hays DM, Kun LE. Solid tumors of childhood. In: DeVita VI, Hellman S, Rosenberg SA, eds. *Cancer: Principles and Practice of Oncology,* 3rd ed. Philadelphia, Pa: JB Lippincott; 1989.

†Leukemia sometimes presents with organomegaly.

ALL=acute lymphocytic leukemia; AML=acute myelogenous leukemia; AMMoL=acute myelomonoblastic leukemia; CML=chronic myelogenous leukemia; MNET=multiple neuroendocrine tumors.

Over the next several years, the relevance of ecogenetics to childhood cancer is expected to become increasingly appreciated.

Leukemias and lymphomas are the most common childhood cancers, accounting for over 40% of cases. Tumors of the central nervous system make up over 20% of childhood malignancies, followed by tumors of the sympathetic nervous system (neuroblastoma), kidney, soft tissues, bone, liver, eye, and germ cells.

BIOLOGY OF CHILDHOOD CANCER

The understanding of the biology and molecular biology of pediatric cancers has exploded in the past decade. The ability to grow tumor cells *in vitro* (in the test tube) and to study their metabolism and the factors that control their growth and differentiation is providing researchers with enormous insights into the basic mechanisms of cancer. The recognition that certain genes (called oncogenes) can transform normal cells into tumor cells has set the stage for understanding the fundamental aspects of tumor formation.

Some cases of childhood malignancies (e.g., retinoblastoma, Wilms' tumor, neuroblastoma) are known to be genetically transmitted. Molecular biology has given researchers the tools to identify specific genes that appear to account for the connection between cancer and genetics. This degree of knowledge may unlock principles that might lead to more selective and effective mechanisms for tumor control and prevention.

A careful evaluation for any genetic basis for malignancy must always be considered in the initial evaluation of the child in whom cancer is diagnosed. Such an evaluation would enable the health care providers to assist the parents with their concerns about future offspring. A careful environmental exposure history should also be taken as part of the overall evaluation of the child with a newly diagnosed malignancy. Environmental factors are increasingly being implicated in the development of tumors in adults, and the possible impact of changes in the environment cannot be overlooked in the pediatric population.

Children with congenital immune deficiency disorders are known to be at increased risk for developing certain malignancies, particularly leukemias and lymphomas. Congenital immunodeficiency diseases, such as ataxia-telangiectasia and Wiskott-Aldrich syndrome, occur infrequently. In the 1990s, however, the number of pediatric patients who are becoming immunodeficient as a consequence of infection with the human immunodeficiency virus (HIV) is expanding rapidly. An increased incidence of lymphomas and other malignancies is being observed in adult patients with acquired immunodeficiency syndrome (AIDS) who are living longer because of improved supportive care and treatments directed against the HIV virus, such as zidovudine (AZT), an antiretroviral drug. As with the adult AIDS population, children with AIDS are benefitting from therapies such as AZT or dideoxyinosine (DDI) that are directed against the primary virus and are expected to live longer and therefore be vulnerable to the development of tumors. The interaction of the immune system in controlling cancer expression thus becomes another piece of the puzzle of how cancer develops and is regulated.

PRINCIPLES OF DIAGNOSIS

The first step in the diagnostic process is to determine whether a cancer is present. This requires using a combination of the child's medical history and physical examination and laboratory measurements, including x-rays and nuclear scans. It is virtually always necessary to perform a biopsy to obtain a tissue sample in order to confirm the diagnosis of cancer.

Because cancer is rare in children, it is not frequently considered in the diagnostic evaluation of a child. Clinical suspicion should be heightened, however, when a child is brought to the physician's office because of the presence of a new mass or lump, unexplained bruising or bleeding, or constitutional symptoms that affect the child's ability to carry on his or her normal activities. These can include fatigue, fever, pallor, weakness, or evidence of lengthy or recurrent infection. Pain at the site of a tumor mass or generalized bone pain due to the invasion of the bone marrow cavities by cancer cells are other signs suggestive of malignancy.

When signs and symptoms suggest a possible malignancy in a child, the first step for the examining pediatrician or physician is to determine how far to proceed with the diagnostic evaluation. If the diagnosis of cancer seems likely, prompt referral to a pediatric oncologist is most appropriate. However, if there is only a suspicion of cancer, further diagnostic evaluation including x-rays, a nuclear scan, and perhaps a biopsy might be undertaken before a referral is made. Once a diagnosis of cancer is confirmed, it is in the best interests of the child and family to assure that treatment will be provided in a center where pediatric cancer specialists and a multidisciplinary team are available to provide the comprehensive care that is necessary to maximize the chances for cure.

STAGING

Even when a tumor appears to be localized to a specific body site, it is highly likely that tumor cells have already spread to distant portions of the body. This process, referred to as micrometastasis, is the rule rather than the exception for nearly all pediatric malignancies. It is important in defining the therapeutic approach. The child undergoing diagnostic evaluation for malignancy should be evaluated extensively to determine the overall extent, or stage of disease, prior to the institution of therapy. Stage defines whether a tumor is localized to its site of origin or whether it has spread to nearby tissues or to more distant organs by the bloodstream or lymphatic channels.

The stage of the disease has important implications for therapy, since tumors that have spread widely require more intensive and longer-duration treatment than localized tumors. Even for localized tumors, the risk for micrometastasis is so great that most children will require treatments that can travel to different parts of the body (such as chemotherapy) in order to eradicate these tumor cell deposits and prevent them from becoming sites of recurrence or relapse. Imaging studies, biological and chemical markers, and cytological and histological diagnostic techniques are useful staging methods.

Imaging Studies

Imaging studies include the use of x-rays, sound waves, magnetism, or radioisotopes to provide an image of a tumor in relationship to the surrounding normal structures. The workhorse in this diagnostic repertoire is the diagnostic radiograph or x-ray. Radiographs provide a two-dimensional view of a body part or structure and provide light and dark contrasts according to the degree of penetration of the x-ray through the body tissue. A chest or a head x-ray is an example of this technique. Although helpful in screening, plain films can miss small tumor deposits. Considerable effort has gone into developing more sophisticated technologies with greater sensitivity and specificity, such as the resolution that results from developing a multidimensional view of a body part. A chest tomogram, for example, provides serial "slices" or images of the lungs and thoracic structures at different levels or depths. This provides a better opportunity to examine the chest cavity as a three-dimensional structure and permits a better localization of a tissue or tumor. Contrast materials, which can enhance or "light up" tumor or surrounding tissues, can be injected into a blood vessel or a body cavity. When combined with a radiographic procedure, it becomes possible to visualize internal structures that would otherwise be indistinct.

A major advance in the ability to visualize the three-dimensional anatomy of the body was the development of computed tomography (CT imaging) during the early 1970s. This technique has revolutionized the staging evaluation of children with cancer. Computed tomography combines x-rays produced from a tube that rotates around the body parts being examined with crystal detectors that convert the x-ray energy into electrical signals. These signals are then analyzed by sophisticated computer programs to construct an intricately detailed image. This detail can be enhanced by the use of contrast material to further highlight specific body parts. The use of CT scanning has allowed the detection of small tumors that might otherwise be invisible. CT imaging can now be done of virtually every body part including the head and brain, sinuses, spinal column, chest, abdomen, pelvis, and extremities. The disadvantages of CT scanning include exposure to x-rays and the need for the child to lie still for an extended period of time. This can be a problem for small children and sedation is often necessary in order to allow the study to be completed. Recently, so-called fast CT scanners have been developed, which may eliminate this problem and provide a new technology with specific application to the imaging of pediatric patients. The procedure is painless, but the scanning apparatus can be intimidating and frightening to a young child. Adequate education and reassurance are intrinsic to the successful completion of these important studies.

During the 1980s, magnetic resonance imaging (MRI) was introduced to clinical use. This technology uses a powerful magnet that stimulates certain atomic nuclei in the body, resulting in the emission of a radio frequency that can be picked up by a receiver. This radio frequency is converted into an electrical signal, which is then processed by sophisticated computer software to create a three-dimensional image of a specific body part. MRI can produce near life-like representations of internal organs and structures, providing the physician with an extraordinary view of body tissues. This is particularly true for images of the brain and spinal cord, but other tissues including muscle can be examined in unparalleled detail. Because tumor tissue produces radiofrequency signals that can differ from those of normal tissue, MRI makes it possible to differentiate between normal and abnormal tissues. Thus, MRI is useful in evaluating localized tumors and assessing potential sites of tumor metastases. An important advantage of MRI is that it provides a means for staging without exposing a patient to additional x-rays. The potential of MRI scans in children is still being evaluated, although this technology represents an important addition to the diagnostic armamentarium.

Ultrasonography is a technique that uses sound waves to develop images of internal organs or body structures. Like MRI, ultrasound (US) is a low-risk, noninvasive procedure. Ultrasound, which is particularly useful for examination of the abdomen and pelvis, is commonly used to evaluate the liver, spleen, kidneys, and retroperitoneum. The disadvantages of US are that the image is not as detailed as that created by CT or MRI and it requires interpretation by trained evaluators.

Radioisotopes can also be used to evaluate the extent of disease. A specific radioisotope is usually injected into a vein, which distributes it throughout the body, and a special detecting camera is used to record the areas where the isotope concentrates. This creates a dotted image of the body or the specific structure that is being examined. Depending upon the isotope and carrier that is used, different body parts can be scanned. For example, technetium permits bone scanning to be accomplished; gallium binds to certain tumors including lymphomas; and the MIBG radioisotope marker is specific for cells that contain neurosecretory granules, such as in neuroblastoma or pheochromocytoma. Isotopes can also be used to measure the energy levels of organs or tumors, a technique referred to as positron emission tomography or PET scanning.

Although each of these techniques can visualize body parts and potential areas of tumor and tumor spread, they do not have the ability to identify actual tumor types. Determining a specific tumor type requires either a specific marker of the tumor or a direct examination of it. Imaging techniques do have a role in this process, however. Biopsies can be performed using fine needles under CT scan guidance, allowing tissue to be obtained without the need for surgery. This technique is being used increasingly in the evaluation of pediatric malignancies.

Biological and Chemical Markers

Certain malignancies secrete biological or chemical substances into the bloodstream or other body fluids (such as urine). These "markers" provide suggestive or inferential evidence of a tumor's presence. For example, neuroblastoma, a tumor of the adrenal glands, may produce elevated levels of catecholamines (e.g., vanillylmandelic acid and homovanillic acid) that are detectable in urine. The presence of these chemicals in conjunction with a clinical picture and imaging analysis suggestive of neuroblastoma further refine the probable diagnosis. The presence of a biological or chemical marker also provides a clue to the burden of disease. Measurements can be taken to determine whether the level of the chemical marker declines when treatment is begun.

Unfortunately, relatively few pediatric tumors produce reliable biological or chemical markers that can be used to stage or follow the course of the malignancy. However, advances in molecular biology may permit the detection of very small amounts of tumor-related materials. Techniques such as the polymerase chain reaction can greatly amplify the presence of a minute quantity of a specific tumor material. The future will likely bring techniques that will permit the ability to diagnose and monitor tumor activity based upon the presence of specific chemical markers in blood, urine, or other body fluids.

PATHOLOGY

The gold standard for diagnosis of a malignancy is the pathological examination, either of cells aspirated from a tumor or from a body fluid in a procedure referred to a cytologic evaluation. Histological examination involves the sectioning of a tumor tissue that was obtained either by biopsy or during a surgical procedure. The thin sections are mounted on glass slides and stained with dyes that provide a contrast of the cellular structure. The specimens are examined in order to define a specific tumor type. Electron microscopy magnifies structures by many thousands and permits detailed examination of cells or even the components of cells. Cytology and histology are the basis for most specific tumor diagnoses in pediatrics.

Bone marrow aspiration is commonly used in the evaluation of many pediatric malignancies, including acute lymphoblastic leukemia (ALL). This procedure involves the insertion of a needle into the inner cavity of a bone, usually of the back or the pelvis, and the aspiration or drawing-up of some of its contents. It is also important in the evaluation of solid tumors that may have spread to the bone marrow.

A bone marrow biopsy involves the use of a special needle to obtain a core of bone and bone marrow. This provides tissue other than just cells that, when sectioned and stained, provide the pathologist with the opportunity to examine the actual architecture of the bone marrow structure. Bone marrow biopsy is also done in the evaluation of acute leukemias, but is especially important in monitoring children with solid tumors. This is because small tumor metastases can become localized and difficult to aspirate and may be detectable only on careful examination of a bone marrow biopsy. Bone marrow biopsies and aspirates can be done safely and easily, but they can be painful. Appropriate education of the child along with local, and sometimes general, sedation are generally necessary.

Histological examination of tumor tissue obtained by surgical or needle biopsy is the major diagnostic procedure for pediatric solid tumors, many of which are commonly referred to as "small blue round cell tumors." Ewing's sarcoma, neuroblastoma, rhabdomyosarcoma, and lymphoma are among this group. Because the histological evaluation can be complicated, a number of sophisticated stains and procedures can be performed on biopsy material. The repertoire of techniques includes electron microscopy, immunocytochemistry, cytogenetics (evaluation of the chromosomes in the cell), and a wide variety of biochemical and molecular biological techniques. Pediatric pathology has become an extraordinarily complex and complicated specialty, but refined diagnoses are increasingly possible.

TUMOR BOARD AND STAGING CONFERENCE

Following the evaluation of the child with suspected cancer, it is imperative that the diagnostic and clinical care specialists meet to review the information that has been collected. This meeting usually takes the form of a tumor board or staging conference in which the pediatric oncologists, surgeons, and radiation therapists meet with the diagnostic radiologists, nuclear medicine specialists, pathologists, and other consultants to review all of the materials that have been obtained. This process enables a specific treatment plan to be developed according to the diagnosis and the extent of the disease. It is also an opportunity to determine whether other procedures might be necessary in order to refine the diagnostic or therapeutic decision making. This forum also guarantees that the child with cancer will benefit from collective expertise of the group and that a plan can be formulated that will provide the greatest opportunity for cure with the lowest chance for unnecessary side effects and morbidity.

PRINCIPLES OF TREATMENT

Once the diagnosis of cancer has been established, the therapeutic plan can be formulated. Although treatment may vary according to the specific nature of the malignancy, a number of principles of therapy are shared among virtually all of the pediatric malignancies. Central to the therapeutic rationale is the fact that pediatric malignancies often grow rapidly, generally spread to various body parts even when undetectable by current diagnostic techniques, and are often sensitive (at least initially) to currently available therapeutic modalities. For patients with solid lesions, such as bone or soft tissue tumors or abdominal masses, local treatment must be determined in addition to the systemic therapy. Local treatment refers to those techniques, primarily surgery and radiation therapy, that will eliminate, eradicate, or attempt to control the primary tumor mass. A child with cancer is also at risk for having systemic disease in addition to a localized tumor mass, so therapy must be administered that can travel to virtually all of the body parts and eradicate undetectable tumor cells. Chemotherapy, or the administration of drugs, is the major modality for providing systemic therapy.

In recent years, biological substances, in some cases materials produced by the body, have been used to enhance or amplify tumor treatment. It is frequently necessary to use two or more modalities together, an approach referred to as multimodal therapy. This concept has revolutionized the treatment of childhood cancer and is largely responsible for the improvements in survival that have been witnessed during recent decades. Although each of the components of multimodal therapy can be used individually and each has specific advantages and disadvantages, they provide a powerful means for tumor control when combined.

Cancer treatment modalities are effective against cancer cells, but they are toxic to normal tissue as well. The prospect for both acute and delayed side effects that can carry serious and incapacitating consequences for the child make it imperative that the treatment be carried out by experienced clinicians who are fully knowledgeable of the benefits and liabilities of each of these powerful modalities. These individuals must be capable of working together as a team to assure that multimodal therapy is carefully integrated into an overall plan that will maximize the child's chances for survival.

SURGERY

Excision or removal of a solid tumor mass is often the first step taken to control a malignancy. For many pediatric malignancies, however, even amputation of a limb can still fail to effect a cure because of the presence of micrometastasis. This not only underscores the importance of adjuvant chemotherapy, but also has lead to a new view of the extent of surgery that should be performed on a growing child. Today, surgical management is guided by two principles. The first is that no child should be considered to have such advanced disease that an attempt at treatment is ruled out. Second, although extensive surgical procedures may sometimes be necessary to control a pediatric malignancy, every attempt should be made to minimize those that have deforming or disabling consequences.

In recent years, a number of revolutionary procedures have been introduced. These include the use of limb-sparing procedures and "neoadjuvant chemotherapy," the latter being the use of anti-cancer drugs to shrink the size of a tumor in order to make it more easily resectable.

Limb-sparing procedures have had a major impact upon the management of bone or soft tissue malignancies. Whereas in the past amputation might have been the only means for tumor removal, limb sparing allows the surgeon to excise tumor-containing bone and tissues and replace it with an artificial prosthesis that allows continued (albeit limited) function of the affected limb. Limb sparing procedures are sophisticated and complicated and must be performed by experienced surgeons. Candidates for limb-sparing must be carefully evaluated. When this procedure is feasible, it can be highly effective in preserving limb function while still providing the opportunity to remove the tumor.

Some large tumors can only be removed by extensive surgical procedures. In some cases the administration of chemotherapy prior to surgery can reduce the size of the tumor to the point where it can be more safely and easily resected. This use of neoadjuvant chemotherapy can, in certain circumstances, allow surgery to be both more successful and more tolerable for children with cancer.

Surgery has another role in cancer treatment. During the past decade, it has become increasingly common for children receiving cancer chemotherapy to have intravenous access devices implanted surgically. These catheters are composed of a soft rubber substance called silastic and, when implanted by a surgeon, permit access to veins for blood sampling and the delivery of chemotherapy. The most frequently used device of this type is the Hickman-Broviac catheter, which is tunneled under the skin of the chest wall, usually exiting around the sternum. Generally, four to eight inches of the catheter extend beyond the skin surface and this extension is usually capped and taped to the chest wall. These catheters are painless to wear and to operate, but they have an impact on the patient's awareness of his or her illness and can cause self-image problems for teenagers who may wish to wear bathing suits. Another type of device is the subcutaneous port, which can be surgically implanted under the skin to serve as a reservoir. Although these devices have the advantage of not being visible from the skin, access to them requires the use of a needle. Both of these surgically implanted devices have significantly improved the quality of life for children undergoing cancer therapy by reducing the number of painful procedures they must endure to receive their treatments.

RADIATION THERAPY

Like surgery, radiation therapy has been a cornerstone of the anti-cancer armamentarium because of its usefulness in local tumor control and in combination regimens. Radiation therapy is a sophisticated science requiring careful planning and simulation to assure that radiation is delivered to the tumor in effective doses, while at the same time sparing surrounding normal tissue. This is particularly important in the pediatric age group in whom radiation therapy can have long-term effects on growth, development, and organ function. It is imperative that children receiving radiation be evaluated in centers where expertise in pediatric radiation therapy is available. As with imaging studies, children undergoing radiation treatments must remain still, to prevent ineffective delivery to the tumor and unnecessary damage to healthy organ tissues. For younger children, generally those younger than 5 years of age, immobilization and sedation are essential components of radiation treatment planning.

Although radiation treatments themselves are painless to receive, higher dose levels can produce uncomfortable skin irritation. The sensitivity of normal tissues to the damaging effects of radiation therapy varies greatly; some organs are relatively resistant and others are exquisitely sensitive. To some degree, sensitivity to radiation depends upon the degree of cell turnover in a specific organ. For example, cells of the skin, mucous membranes, gonads, and the hematopoietic (blood forming) system are very sensitive to the effects of radiation therapy because of their high multiplication rates.

A general goal of radiation treatment is to encompass the entire tumor within the radiation field while sparing as much normal tissue as possible. In some cases, radiation therapy is delivered to the entire body as part of a preparative regimen for bone marrow transplantation, a procedure referred to as total body irradiation (TBI). This form of radiation therapy has a significant impact upon the hematopoietic and immunological systems, and this effect can be fatal if reconstitution is not accomplished by bone marrow transplantation. Like chemotherapy, total body irradiation is a form of systemic therapy because radiation is administered to virtually all areas of the body.

CHEMOTHERAPY

More than any other anti-cancer treatment modality, chemotherapy has had a pivotal role in improving survival. Chemotherapy drugs are referred to as cytotoxic agents because they result in cell death. These compounds may act on a cell during a particular cycle, or may be effective regardless of the stage of a tumor cell's development. Some of these drugs act by interfering with the cell's genes or DNA, others with its RNA, while others interrupt protein synthesis. Regardless of the exact mechanism of action, the common thread is that the tumor cell is rendered unable to carry on its functions of growth and reproduction.

Chemotherapeutic agents may favor the destruction of tumor cells that are multiplying, but they are also capable of causing similar damage to normal body tissues that are also multiplying and dividing. This is the reason that the administration of chemotherapy is associated with so many side effects and sequelae. Normal tissue with high cell turnover rates are most susceptible to the adverse affects of chemotherapy. Thus, common side effects associated with chemotherapy include hair loss, nausea and vomiting, sores in the mouth and gastrointestinal tract, and suppression of the bone marrow. Each of these side effects has an impact upon the pediatric cancer patient and family. Hair loss can be devastating to adolescents, because it will make them feel and look different from their peers at a time in their life when appearance is so important to self-esteem. Mouth sores can be painful and can affect the child's ability to eat and maintain proper nutrition. Suppression of the bone marrow can be life-threatening. In light of potential side effects, chemotherapy schedules must be carefully designed and monitored. Accordingly, children receiving chemotherapy should be cared for in centers that have expertise in pediatric oncology. It is also important for the child and family to understand both the beneficial effects and side effects of chemotherapy and to become partners in the care and support necessary to sustain the treatment program.

Most schedules include combinations of agents. This approach maximizes the activity of the regimen by using agents that work in different manners, thereby taking advantage of their additive effects in the destruction of tumor cells. Combination regimens also minimize the ability of cancer cells to escape destruction by having developed resistance to a particular drug. Usually, chemotherapy regimens are administered in cycles, often on a monthly basis, to give the patient adequate time to recover from treatment effects and lessen the buildup of toxicity.

The immediate goal of chemotherapy is to produce a remission of the cancer; that is, all measurable components of the cancer have been eliminated. Remission does not mean that all the cancer has been eradicated, because many tumor cells can be present in the body and yet escape detection by even the most sophisticated technologies. Chemotherapy is often administered over many months, and in some diseases over years, to maintain control of the malignancy. During this period of maintenance therapy, the goal is to continue reducing the body's tumor burden with the ultimate goal of eradicating it and thus producing a cure.

Investigational Principles

Tumors vary in their sensitivities to various cytotoxic drugs, and it is by trial-and-error that physicians have ascertained which agents are most active against a particular malignancy. The evaluation of investigational agents is critical to future success in the treatment of children with cancer. Three phases are followed in the evaluation of chemotherapeutic agents. Phase I testing involves the assessment of safety and tolerance of a new agent and is basically designed to determine the dose that can be tolerated. In general, Phase I testing does not begin in children until testing has proceeded in adults. The development of therapeutic agents for children with HIV infection, however, has forced a reconsideration of this policy. It is anticipated that the pace of drug development for children with cancer might also be accelerated as a consequence of these insights. Once a dosage of a chemotherapeutic agent has been found to be safe and tolerable, the agent then undergoes Phase II testing, in which its activity against different tumor types is determined. The tumors that might be most likely to respond to a new chemotherapeutic agent can be discerned in part from the results of testing in experimental *in vitro* systems as well as in animal experiments. If a drug appears to be active in Phase II testing against a specific tumor, it is then ready for Phase III trials in which its activity is compared to known agents. In general, Phase I testing requires only a small number of patients to ascertain safety, tolerance, and dose findings. Phase II testing might require 25 to 100 or more patients. Phase III comparative studies generally involve hundreds or thousands of patients.

Comparative assessment using randomized clinical trials is an essential component of drug development. It is the only way to avoid bias and assure the activity of a new agent. A new drug or a combination of drugs is assessed within the context of a protocol that spells out the exact details of the regimen to be studied and allows the data to be accrued in a way that accurate interpretation is assured. Because pediatric malignancies are uncommon, many of the protocols conducted in the United States are done as part of multi-institutional studies, in which centers around the country collaborate and cooperate to evaluate new treatment concepts or to fine-tune those that have already become established. Most of these cooperative trials are performed under the auspices of the Pediatric Oncology Group and the Children's Cancer Study Group. These groups, supported by the National Cancer Institute, have been successfully enrolling about 60% of children with cancer into clinical protocols. By assuring that as many children as possible are being enrolled in state-of-the-art treatment protocols, the prospect exists for improving the outcome for future children with cancer.

Chemotherapy Administration Principles

Chemotherapeutic agents are generally administered orally or intravenously. In some protocols, agents are administered into the artery (intra-arterial chemotherapy) to deliver therapy to a specific tumor site. Certain chemotherapeutic agents, including vincristine, daunorubicin, and doxorubicin, can cause considerable damage if they infiltrate or extravasate out of the vein. This problem is largely avoided by the use of Hickman-Broviac catheters.

Because cancer cells can survive in areas of the body in which chemotherapy has limited access (e.g., the central nervous system [CNS]), it is sometime necessary to deliver the agents into the spinal fluids. This intrathecal therapy is integral to the treatment of several childhood cancers, most notably leukemias and lymphomas, and is a component of CNS prophylaxis.

It is an important aspect of pediatric cancer care that all members of the patient's health care team be aware of the range of potential side effects so that appropriate support for the patient can be given. Some of these treatment modalities carry delayed or chronic toxic effects in addition to acute side effects. For example, during or shortly after administration of chemotherapeutic agents, patients may experience nausea and vomiting because of the drug's impact on the trigger zones in the areas of the brain that control the vomiting reflex. Antiemetic medications can suppress this reaction. Nausea and vomiting represent an uncomfortable treatment side effect, but the occurrence of hair loss and mouth sores represent both the stigmata of cancer treatment as well as sources of pain and discomfort. Depending upon the child's preferences, the hair loss can be creatively masked by scarves or wigs and the mouth sores aided by good oral hygiene. Chemotherapy-related bone marrow suppression, however, represents a true limitation of treatment because all three components of the blood cells can be suppressed as a consequence of cancer treatment. Depleted red blood cells and platelets are treatable with either packed red blood cells or platelet transfusions, thereby allowing therapy to continue. Also, modifying the dosage and frequency of the chemotherapy can attenuate some of these marrow-related side effects. Suppression of the white blood cells, however, constitutes a major problem for both the child and the medical care staff. A white blood count that falls to low levels, particularly when it remains low for days to weeks at a time, increases the risk for developing a life-threatening infection. Most of the organisms that contribute to these infections are endogenous, arising from the body's own microbiological flora. In the absence of the body's defending cells, these organisms can result in serious infections. In a child undergoing cancer therapy, any sign of infection, particularly when the white blood cell count is low, should be immediately brought to the attention of the child's physician. Any fever in conjunction with a low white blood cell count is reason for immediate evaluation and almost certainly will result in the child's admission to the hospital for intravenous antibiotic therapy. This approach of quick response to signs of infection has largely overcome the life-threatening sequelae associated with low blood counts and infection. This points out the need to include the parents and the child, when appropriate, as part of the health care team so that they are well educated about the adverse effects of therapy and, in particular, when to call for help.

Many of the therapeutic effects and side effects of chemotherapy are directly related to the intensity or the amount of therapy that is being administered. Intensity is either a high dose of a drug or combination of drugs administered at any point in time, or the very frequent administration of chemotherapeutic agents. Generally, more intensive chemotherapy regimens are associated with a greater degree of therapeutic effects and side effects. Situations occur in which high-dose chemotherapy regimens are essential in order to provide the maximum chances for survival, as in the treatment of acute leukemias or high-risk solid tumors. In these situations, very high doses of chemotherapy may be necessary to provide the maximum degree of tumor cell eradication.

Perhaps the most extreme examples of this are the regimens used in bone marrow transplantation, which in the past decade became an important component of childhood cancer treatment. Bone marrow transplantation was first established for the treatment of children with leukemia, and subsequently for lymphoma, and has more recently been used in the treatment of a number of solid-tumor malignancies. Bone marrow transplantation is a reconstitution or rescue regimen. The major strategy is to be able to deliver the highest possible dosage of chemotherapy and other modalities, such as radiation therapy, in order to have the greatest impact on the tumor. Because such intensive therapy can result in profound suppression of the bone marrow for very long periods of time, the administration of bone marrow might hasten the patient's recovery and attenuate some of these toxic side effects. The experience gained during the last decade has demonstrated that bone marrow transplantation can reconstitute the marrow in patients who have received very high dose regimens.

There are two sources of bone marrow that can be administered to patients. Autologous bone marrow is the patient's own bone marrow, harvested at a time when the disease is in remission, often treated to eradicate any residual cells, and frozen and stored until it is administered back to the patient. With allogeneic bone marrow transplantation, the source of the marrow is someone other than the patient. The best source of an allogeneic bone marrow transplantation donor is a sibling or family member of the patient. During recent years, a number of registries have been developed so that persons unrelated to the patient whose marrow might be compatible with the patient can be identified as possible donors.

Transplantation of bone marrow can be successful in the treatment of acute leukemias in particular, but it is still best to view bone marrow transplantation as an investigational procedure for many of the other pediatric malignancies. It is essential that these procedures are performed at centers that are equipped to deal with children who undergo a bone marrow transplant.

BIOLOGICAL THERAPIES

The advances in molecular biology and recombinant DNA technology made it possible during the 1980s to generate large quantities of molecules that serve as chemical signals affecting the body's immune and hematopoietic systems. Among these agents are cytokines, a generic term for nonantibody proteins released by certain types of cells on contact with a specific antigen. These act as intercellular mediators, as in generating an immune response. Agents known as the granulocyte-macrophage-colony stimulating factor (GM-CSF) or granulocyte-colony stimulating factor (G-CSF) both appear to be capable of accelerating the time to bone marrow recovery following the administration of cytotoxic chemotherapy. The integration of these "biologicals" into chemotherapy schedules may lessen some of the side effects, in particular reducing the duration of low white blood cell counts (neutropenia) and the associated risk for developing serious infections. Studies evaluating these biologicals in children with cancer are under way, and it is anticipated that their role in the treatment of pediatric malignancies will be discerned within the next several years. Cytokines eventually may play a pivotal role in the care of children with cancer by both decreasing toxicity and enhancing the tumoricidal activity of chemotherapy.

The interleukins and the interferons are other molecules that may play an important role in the treatment of malignancy or in the supportive care of pediatric cancer patients. These agents are being evaluated in children and their role in combination regimens should be discerned within the next several years. The ability to use the immune system as part of cancer treatment has been demonstrated in several adult malignancies, particularly renal cell cancer and melanoma. A strategy combining the administration of interleukin 2 with lymphokine activated killer cells has been shown to exert an impressive effect in some adult malignancies. Additional strategies being explored in adults include the use of tumor infiltrating lymphocytes, which may be more specific in their destruction of a tumor. These adoptive immunotherapy regimens have only begun to be explored in children, but they may play an increasing role in the future. Studies to evaluate tumor infiltrating lymphocyte cell therapy for neuroblastoma, for example, are under way at the National Cancer Institute.

FUTURE CONSIDERATIONS IN PEDIATRIC CANCER TREATMENT

The major goal in the treatment of the child with cancer is to utilize therapies that are specific for the tumor and that spare the child as much toxicity as possible. The evolving understanding of the molecular basis of cancer may well facilitate the ability to treat pediatric malignancies by novel mechanisms. In addition to the application of biologicals, it may be possible to reprogram tumors to differentiate and to stop multiplying, thus rendering them incapable of spreading locally or metastasizing to other parts of the body. Insights gained from *in vitro* studies suggest that a number of chemical agents and biological agents may be useful in accomplishing this cellular reprogramming, and further work is expected. If successful, these strategies could further improve the impact of cancer treatment as well as enhance the quality of life of the children who receive treatment for the disease.

PRINCIPLES OF THE MULTIDISCIPLINARY APPROACH TO CARING FOR CHILDREN WITH CANCER

When malignancy is suspected in a child, many resources and technologies must be integrated in order to determine whether a cancer exists, the nature of a primary cancer that is diagnosed, and the extent to which the disease may have spread prior to the initiation of therapy. This comprehensive assessment requires the expertise of pediatric oncologists, surgeons, radiation therapists and radiologists, nuclear medicine specialists, pathologists, and cytologists. All play intricate roles in the overall evaluation of the child with probable or proven cancer. Once the diagnosis is established, cancer treatment requires the integration of many resources and skills to maximize the child's chance of survival and minimize the toxic effects of treatment that might ensue. Skilled physicians and nurses form the base of the medical therapeutic alliance. However, treatment without the psychosocial support and care of the child and his or her family would be incomplete. Thus, essential members of the multidisciplinary team also include social workers, psychologists, physical and occupational therapists, recreational therapists, teachers, and members of the clergy. Each contributes insight, care, and understanding to the child with cancer. Many therapies must be administered in a hospital or outpatient clinic, so interruption of family life cannot be avoided. As much attention as possible must be given to helping the pediatric cancer patients and their families lead as normal lives as are possible. Part of this supportive approach is to help the child remain in school and look forward to the prospect of successful treatment and even cure. Contact with schools and community services represents an arm of the cancer treatment program that requires the assistance of the multidisciplinary team.

It is estimated that in the 1990s, 1 of every 1000 young people between the ages of 18 and 25 will be a cancer survivor. Clearly, although a number of these young people will have been cured of their underlying disease, they will also have experienced side effects related to treatment. Whether these include impaired growth, sterility, heart problems, or physical limitations, it is important to learn from the experiences of children who have survived cancer treatment, and thus to develop even better treatment strategies in the future.

SUGGESTED READING

Further information on the subject of diagnosis and treatment of cancer in children can be found in the text *Principles and Practice of Pediatric Oncology,* 2nd ed. Pizzo PA and Poplack DG, eds. Philadelphia Pa: JB Lippincott; 1992.

UNDERSTANDING THE FAMILY EXPERIENCE WITH CHILDHOOD CANCER

Judith W. Ross, MSW, ACSW, LISW

FACTORS AFFECTING FAMILY RESPONSE TO A CHILDHOOD CANCER DIAGNOSIS

Despite impressive progress that prolongs lives and cures many, a diagnosis of pediatric cancer is received with fear and dread. Aside from the disease, patients, parents, and other family members experience a complex array of social, emotional, economic, and familial stresses that have their roots in the structure of our society and the roles assigned to parents and children.

Characteristics such as smaller family size, insulated nuclear units, and prolonged dependence of offspring upon their parents create special vulnerabilities for each member of modern Western families. Society places high expectations on parents, who are responsible for their children's behavior, appearance, and health. When a child is struck with so serious an illness as cancer, parents often respond with feelings of guilt and a sense of having failed in their exclusive responsibilities. The special obligations and extraordinary emotional bonds between parents and their children, as well as the vulnerability and dependency of children, define parent-child relationships as unique in society. Therefore, childhood cancer "represents an assault on a parent's sense of adequacy as a guardian of his child."[1] These aspects make childhood cancer a special case, related to but distinct from the experiences and issues that surround cancer in adults.

Most children with cancer are treated at specialized cancer centers to which they have been referred. Although parents may have been forwarned by a pediatrician, family doctor, or a physician from the local hospital of the seriousness of their child's illness and the possible (or probable) diagnosis of cancer, they are considerably stressed and worried regardless of how well they may have been prepared. Many factors interact to influence parents' initial and subsequent responses to hospital staff members, to questions posed, to medical and bureaucratic procedures, and to the barrage of information presented to them. In addition, parents must respond to the larger concerns and issues created by their child's illness.

The psychosocial aspects of childhood cancer can be understood in terms of phases. Cancer itself has characteristic phases: diagnosis, remission, exacerbation, and survival or terminal periods. Similarly, treatment is divided into phases: induction, intensification, consolidation, and maintenance. Each phase of illness and treatment challenges the family and patient.

CRISIS RESPONSES

Experts and family members often refer to the time of diagnosis as a crisis. Crisis theory provides a framework for considering parental response during this period. According to this theory, people generally have a need for social and psychological equilibrium or maintenance of a "steady state." When they "encounter something that upsets their balance, habitual problem-solving mechanisms are employed until the balance is restored."[2] A diagnosis of cancer in child presents "a situation that is so novel, so major that the habitual responses are inadequate... (this) constitutes a crisis and leads to a state of disorganization often accompanied byanxiety, fear, guilt, or other unpleasant feelings which contribute further to the disorganization."[3]

The negative connotations of the disease, derived from its association with death and unhappy memories of stricken relatives or friends[4], contribute to the crisis atmosphere. The fear and distress evoked by the threat of death and suffering and the uncertainty regarding outcome combine to make the time of diagnosis inordinately stressful. Parents realize that their child's life is in jeopardy and that the family faces enormous, irreversible, and unforeseeable changes. Immediate and future expectations and cherished hopes and plans for the child and the family unit are at risk. Self concept, esteem, confidence, sense of independence, and autonomy are threatened. Parents are unable to predict or to control the course of events; they cannot protect their child, themselves, and others in the family. At a time when they are feeling vulnerable and experiencing emotional turmoil, parents are being exposed to complex and unfamiliar information that they find difficult to translate into meaningful and predictable terms. Crisis theory helps to explain parental behavior during this early phase of the illness and at other points of stress through delineation of several major adaptive tasks.[2] These tasks are a complex set of responses to the illness that result in practical or psychological activities accomplished through the use of coping skills.[2,5] The parents' realization that their child may die is an example of a psychological task associated with the diagnostic phase of the illness. Other tasks are informing family, considering what and how to tell the patient about the illness, arranging for the care of other children, evaluating their financial resources, and fulfilling other responsibilities.

This is the family's task:

> They now come to focus on themselves as parents of a seriously ill child. The other members of the family confront similiar tasks. As they grapple with these tasks, they are developing psychosocial 'tools,' mechanisms for surmounting stress. These tools, acquired during each phase of the illness, are necessary to resolve the stress of the next phase. When there is a failure to develop such tools, each successive phase of the illness is experienced as if it were the first and the obstacles to adaptive coping may be compounded.[5]

Other challenges to the steady state are related to specific aspects of the illness, such as the child's discomfort level and prognosis. Among parental tasks are receiving and integrating information; managing feelings of guilt, fear, and anxiety; forming relationships with health care staff; and supporting their child. The child's tasks will be determined largely by age and stage of development. In order to accomplish these diverse tasks, parents must achieve a delicate balance between grasping the gravity of the situation and remaining hopeful of a positive outcome. This requires a certain amount of minimizing, sometimes called denial.

Childhood cancer therapy is extremely complex, usually involving a combination of surgery, chemotherapy, and/or radiation therapy, performed or delivered in specialized centers. Most children are treated according to predetermined treatment plans, or protocols, which seek to improve understanding of cancers and their treatment. The diagnostic tests, methods of delivering treatment, unfamiliar and strange-sounding names of chemotherapy agents, roadmaps, confusing schedules, and frequent monitoring of blood counts and heart, kidney, and liver functions all contribute to making the parents of a child with cancer feel overwhelmed. The fear that their child will be a guinea pig adds to their stress.

Parents need to understand the medical facts being presented to them in order to make appropriate decisions and grant permission for diagnostic or therapeutic procedures, yet they must also regulate or control the amount of information they receive to avoid becoming immobilized by facts. Information has the potential to overwhelm, but it can also help parents (and the patient and siblings as well) feel more in control. When the patient and family know what to expect and understand what is taking place the medical universe and the events occurring within it have less power to frighten them. At first, information is provided to them; eventually, they can seek answers to specific questions and gain knowledge through experience and observation. Parents who manage their emotions create energy reserves for performing practical and affective tasks, including providing comfort and support to the patient and to the other members of the family. Parents who are burdened by guilt, paralyzed by fear, and unable to be consoled or to find hope may not be able to learn how to care for their child at home. Self-mastery protects each individual, strengthens the sense of self, and facilitates the necessary adjustments in life-style and roles. Parents who remain calm can reassure their child and help him or her face discomfort and the unknown.

Inability to form connections with staff extends the sense of crisis. Parents who cannot trust, reach out to, or respond to overtures from professional caregivers may be at great risk for dysfunction. Positive relationships formed with caretaking staff can increase the family's sense of hope.

Each of these crisis-induced behaviors is a positive coping strategy, but each also has the potential to be maladaptive. If, for example, the parents regulate the amount of information they receive to the extent that they are ignorant about side effects of treatment or other potential complications or otherwise unprepared to manage care at home, their ability to make appropriate judgments and to safeguard their child is impaired. Parents who do not respond to signs or symptoms of illness or who are overvigilant and perceive medical catastrophes with minimal provocation may lack the integrated information necessary to make appropriate assessments of their child's well being. Too much control over emotions can interfere with an individual's ability to work through fears and worries, thus resulting in overaccumulation of delayed reactions, inappropriate or unpredictable displays of anger, anxiety, depression, and an inability to respond to current situations.

Children are exquisitely attuned to their fathers and mothers and their sense of and response to the crisis is deeply influenced by the parents' reactions. Despite parents' efforts to control their emotions, the child is aware of subtle changes in mood, demeanor, and touch. Children respond to and feel protected by positive cues from parents and reasonable explanations and preparation for medical events. The physical effects of illness, combined with the unfamiliar and intimidating surroundings and examinations and other contact by unfamiliar people, contribute to the child's sense of crisis. Preteens and adolescents have the intellectual capacity to permit a comprehensive explanation of the medical problem. However, these age groups have an increased sense of awareness of the possibility of permanent disability and death that can heighten their fears.[6] Children in crisis exhibit a broad range of behaviors. They may become irritable, demanding, cranky, aggressive, hyperactive, withdrawn, uncommunicative, or passive.

FAMILY CHARACTERISTICS

The young cancer patient must be understood in the context of his or her family, which provides the framework for the major adjustments made by the child. Successful adaptation to arduous treatment and the changes brought about in appearance, stamina, and sense of well being depends on how members of the family respond to the illness and to the child. A child who is accepted by the family will be able to withstand the adverse reactions of others.[4]

Each family is unique in its character and history; internal and external relationships; cultural, religious, and ethnic background; and in other attributes, all of which interact to create a functional or dysfunctional system. This system is not static; family members (and the unit itself) are capable of extensive growth and change that often surprise even themselves. These changes may be stimulated by subtle alterations in one individual or by catastrophic events. Social workers who meet parents of a child being evaluated for possible malignancy may have difficulty seeing them as leaders of a healthy, working family unit if they exhibit extremes of behavior and demeanor. For the most part, families who were successful prior to onset of a child's illness are likely to make the adjustments necessary for continued if not optimal functioning.

The flexibility to adjust their priorities, an ability to use outside supports, resourcefulness in anticipating and formulating needs, and growth throughout the critical phases of the illness are hallmarks of successful family coping. "Few families are absolutely devoid of strengths, but some may be so distracted or incapacitated by past problems or current dysfunctions in their relationships that they are unable to mobilize their resources to adjust to the crisis of a child with cancer."[7]

There are some families for whom the illness, because of its nature or its timing, poses a challenge that cannot be met without major changes. In such cases both individual members and the family unit are at risk and the young patients are overburdened with additional stresses. Visits from parents and other family members cannot be anticipated, nor their support assured, so the child is often alone during medical procedures and comfort for the accompanying trauma must come from staff. Other families cope well with the extraordinary demands of the illness but are unable to return to more normal styles of functioning once the crisis is passed.

A child's illness creates a need for the parents to share decisions and responsibilities, but unremitting conflicts can make sharing impossible. A marriage may be unworkable, dissolving, or involve uneasy truces replete with rigid or unshifting rules and roles that can only change with the most painstaking negotiations.[7] Marital problems can distract the mother and father from their responsibilities as parents and deplete emotional resources needed to help the patient and siblings.

Answers to specific questions can provide a perspective for understanding each particular family and the nature and intensity of assistance they will need. First, who are the members of the family? Is it a two-parent home where father and mother love and support one another? Or do they lead separate, isolated, or circumscribed lives? Are the parents separated, divorced, remarried, or never married? What is their relationship with each other and with the patient? Can they put aside differences for their own and the child's sake? Or will they use this occasion to tear one another down, revive or aggravate long-standing differences and bitterness? A lack of mutual support at a time of increased need results in misunderstanding, isolation, and aggravated tension for parents and the children.[7]

Do the parents conform to rigid role expectations? Or are they flexible and open to adjustments that will enhance and benefit each member, while caring for the special needs of the sick child and maintaining a sense of family unity? Besides the patient, are there other family members who are vulnerable as a result of physical illness or emotional, behavioral, or school problems? Is there alcohol or drug abuse, gambling, or other compulsive, antisocial, or criminal behavior? Are the emotional and adaptive resources already strained because of problems of other members of the family and/or significant associates? Escalating problems of other troubled members can lead to unmanageable behavior that impedes or distracts the caretakers from dealing with the necessary tasks.

What is the life stage of the family? Is it a young family with a couple learning how to be parents and establish independence from their own families of origin? Or is this an older family with most of the other children grown and away from the home, the parents looking forward to more freedom with the departure of the one who has now become ill? The issues confronting parents who have nearly completed child-rearing and are anticipating retirement are distinctly different from the issues faced by a young couple whose first child has become ill with a life-threatening disease.

Developmental factors influence the way the child and the parents experience the illness and interact with one another. Feelings and concerns evoked in parents differ depending on whether they have an infant with a serious medical problem or a seriously ill adolescent. What is the age and birth order of the patient, and how will his or her illness affect the hopes and plans of the other members?[3] Have the parents and other siblings doted on the youngster to the extent that self-discipline was never expected or developed? Will the patient find inner resources to endure unpleasant and painful treatment and maintain important peer relationships? Or is this a child who already has experienced educational, emotional, or other adjustment problems that will interact negatively with the new demands created by the illness?

Has the illness occurred at a time when other significant changes are occurring: mother returning to work, new baby arrived or expected, father out of work, family recently relocated or planning to move, other close relatives ill or recently deceased? Even positive changes produce stress that can contribute to parents' sense of being overwhelmed.

What has been the family's previous experience with crisis or illness? Are parents likely to feel defeated by the child's problem, or will they take strength from jointly having met other challenges successfully?

What are the patterns of communicating information, feelings, and ideas? Can fears be expressed, talked through, and resolved? Can individual members tolerate exposure to one another's emotional pain? What content and level of emotional responses are permitted or valued?[3] Although parental partners may care for each other and manage the day-to-day responsibilities of their lives, they may be unpracticed in communicating to each other their needs and feelings.[7] Voicing feelings is more difficult in times of extreme stress and parents often expect more of each other and of their children during crisis. Their expectations escalate, yet they may not be shared with their partners and may be based on unrealistic appraisals of what spouses or others in the family are capable of.

Are parents and/or children impulsive, emotionally labile, peseverating? Is there a history of family violence? Or are family members passive, withdrawn, and unable to express feelings? Parents who are inaccessible because of uncommunicative or explosive styles typically are unable to offer appropriate support to the patient and often pose problems for staff.

What is the nature of the parent-child relationship? Is the patient closer to one parent? Are the parents realistic in their expectations of children, or are they unable to discipline, overly permissive, or unduly strict? Are generational boundaries intact, or are children parentified (i.e., permitted to assume a parent's role)? Adaptive capacities can be strained by the illness, causing the relationship between the parents and the child to deteriorate. Parents tend to be exceedingly solicitous of the child at the time of diagnosis and while they await remission of the disease, but prolonged solicitude and special treatment can have a deleterious effect on the child's behavior. If discipline is lacking and pampering continues long after the child is discharged from the hospital and is feeling well, changes in the parents' attitudes will alarm the child. In response, the child may act in a way that cries out for limits and the security of accustomed parental control. However, the parents may not be sufficiently attuned to the child's needs. If they are depressed and enervated by the illness, or without hope concerning prognosis, they may lose sight of what their present behavior tells the child about his or his future. Unaccustomed and inappropriate power over the parents may evoke fear, anger or tyrannical behavior in the child. Or, the child may cling to the parents and regress to an earlier, safer period of development.[7]

Regression does not always indicate dysfunction in the parent-child relationship. Children often cope with the trauma of physical illness by temporarily regressing; a child who was toilet trained may have accidents, or one who walked may demand to be carried. In younger children disruption of milestones is easy to document, but older children may exhibit more subtle effects. With encouragement and reassurance the child often regains previous skills, but often parents are distressed by regression and need to be instructed regarding how to interpret and handle such behavior when it occurs.

What is the patient's place in the family? Before the illness was the child considered special in some way that will influence how he or she is considered now? Has the patient already been the recipient of more than the usual share of parental love? Do the siblings regard the renewed attention as adding insult to injury?

The sibling of a child with cancer is in an exquisite double bind. He or she must attempt to reconcile the opposing strong feelings associated with the combination of sibling love and profound resentment. The brother or sister is caught between a need to be like and associated with the one who is ill, while also wanting and needing to be separate and an individual. A sibling can recognize how parents' hopes and dreams, once focused on all the children, now seem to reside in the fate of one particular child. A sibling's own need and desire for parental love and attention is moderated by feelings of guilt and shame.

Sibling identity is closely interconnected. A child cannot be a big brother without a younger sibling or a little sister without an older sibling.[8] Mingled self-consciousness further complicates the sibling's plight, but siblings hesitate to express feelings to parents for fear of further alienation and rejection, or because they know that to voice such thoughts would not be acceptable. Parents usually expect more of older siblings, who often are given more responsibility for household tasks and for child care and are more likely to be expected to forgo their own desires and plans.

If there are no other children in the family, the parents are faced with the terrifying possibility of not being parents at all should the child die. The parents' sense of who they are as individuals as well as the ties between them as a couple are threatened when the cancer patient is an only child.

Grandparents may offer comfort, support, respite, moral and personal reinforcement, and practical assistance, or they can be critical, blaming, and withholding of material and emotional aid. Relationships between adult children and their parents vary considerably. Problems may be forgotten in response to the crisis, or they may become worse and create additional strain. Grandparents who are emotionally or physically fragile can distract from the needs of the young patient and nuclear family. Just as the parents either provide the patient with ways to accept and deal with the illness or fail to do so, the grandparents can be reaffirming or can thwart the efforts of the patient and parents to adjust.

Spiritual, religious, and philosophical beliefs can add considerable strength to a family's ability to accept and cope with adversity. Such beliefs can also shield an individual from assuming self-blame and guilt. Parents who accept their child's illness as part of a greater cosmic or spiritual plan or who expect to be reunited in an afterlife often can accept the illness and its possible negative outcome with more composure than those parents who have no such belief system.

Social support is another important ingredient of coping. The observation that parents who solicit, receive, and accept emotional and practical support from family, friends, and members of the community are greatly bolstered and in turn can be helpful to the patient and siblings is well documented. Parents whose need to maintain control is expressed by rejecting or withdrawing from supportive contacts may suffer painful isolation. Friends and family can mediate stress, give needed relief from a bedside vigil, care for siblings, perform household tasks such as laundry or meals, or provide transportation. Social workers can assist families in accepting such resources.

At times, a social worker's early interactions with parents suggest that there are unresolved conflicts, residual developmental issues, or responses that were more appropriate to past crises. For parents who are extremely passive, angry, or who seem to be rebelling against perceived authority, the diagnosis of cancer, the hospitalization, the painful procedures, or some other aspect of their child's illness evokes emotions and behavior that hail from other, previous, or more fundamental problems. Lessening of the parents' stress in some cases may encourage greater control over behavior even though it will not resolve the problem. In other instances, serious psycho- or sociopathology warrants more intensive, comprehensive intervention. Social workers should be aware of the vast range of normal responses to a crisis such as that precipitated by cancer. Even families whose behavior appears unusually extreme may regroup and achieve a level of preillness, adaptive functioning that will allow the patient to be nurtured and receive medical care and the other family members to receive accustomed attention. Inexperienced professional caregivers should avoid forming premature opinions or expecting too much too soon from families who, given time, can function at an acceptable level.

In most pediatric centers, social workers are integral members of the treatment team and, as such, meet all families. This practice is especially advantageous with families whose serious problems predate the child's illness because it permits formation of routine and trusting relationships that can accommodate a directive approach to focus attention on these issues. Counseling may be offered at the treatment center or through referral to another provider. When team collaboration is not the norm, the social worker will face some special challenges addressing family needs. With all families, understanding their responses in the early stages and providing guidance and support can do much to prevent or lessen future problems.

ILLNESS FACTORS AND DEVELOPMENTAL ISSUES

EVENTS SURROUNDING DIAGNOSIS

A diagnosis of cancer usually bears no relationship to a child's previous health status. Most children who develop cancer were previously healthy. Regardless of the child's age, initial symptoms can be similar to those of ordinary childhood illness and consequently do not alarm parents or pediatricians. Many forms of childhood malignancy, such as Wilms' tumor, are discovered during a routine visit to the doctor. Certain forms of leukemia may produce symptoms without making the child appear ill.

In such instances it may be difficult for parents to accept that their child is sick, particularly with so serious a medical problem. Within a matter of hours, parents who had no reason to suspect that their child's life was in danger may be confronted with decisions about surgery or other invasive medical procedures. Informed of the potential for adverse or even fatal side effects from treatment or for a negative outcome, parents may react with understandable shock, disbelief, fear, helplessness, grief, and hostility depending upon previous experiences or temperament.

Anger, distrust, self-blame, and other strong emotions can be evoked and complicate what is, at best, a devastating experience if parents who were convinced that something was wrong with their child received inadequate, off-putting, patronizing, or other minimizing responses from previously trusted or respected physicians. Similar emotions may be displayed if symptoms were misunderstood, the medical work-up was mismanaged, or the child's complaints were attributed to malingering or to emotional disturbance and progression of disease or impairment resulted.

Even in the most enlightened pediatric cancer center, pinpointing the diagnosis is not invariably straightforward, as many childhood cancers are associated with primitive, undifferentiated body tissue. Delays in arriving at a conclusive diagnosis and definitive treatment plan prolong uncertainty, thus aggravating the parents' already escalated level of stress and strained emotional resources.

If the child arrives at the treatment facility already ill-appearing, in distress from pain or respiratory, cardiac, or renal compromise, or with other potentially fatal complications, the parents' focus will be on the imminent threat to the child's life. The immediate crisis must ease before parents can be expected to grasp the overall implications of the disease. What parents are told and what they understand about their child's prognosis will also influence them in the first few weeks of the diagnostic period. If the serious nature of the disease is trivialized because of an extremely hopeful prognosis and relatively mild treatment protocol, the parents will be understandably positive. On the other hand, parents who are given no hope for their child's extended survival may have difficulty even considering therapy.

Parental adjustment also depends upon the severity of the disease and the child's initial response, in terms of ability to tolerate therapy and the resolution of symptoms, as well as upon their own perceptions of their child's reactions. Parents who regard the treatment as more dangerous or less tolerable than the illness will find it difficult to encourage their child to comply with the recommended course. In some cases, the treatment and the medical personnel who prescribe and deliver it become villains from whom the parents feel they must rescue their child.

THE CHILD'S RESPONSE TO TREATMENT

Certain childhood cancers are congenital, others occur in the first months or years of life. Several of these have high cure rates, but other cancers that affect infants often do not respond to treatment and length of survival is limited. Parents of seriously ill infants have distinctive emotional burdens. In addition to not being able to protect their child from painful medical interventions, they cannot explain what has happened, nor can they prepare the infant for what will come. Infants cannot communicate the location or extent of physical pain or the nature of their apprehensions and fears, so fathers and mothers can only observe the baby's reactions and imagine the baby's thoughts. Adults, particularly parents, are deeply affected by the suffering of an infant; mothers of babies with cancer suffer intensely because of the close biological tie between mothers and their babies. One consolation is that fathers and mothers may also be extremely close during the days, weeks, and months following a baby's birth and can take strength from each other and their relationship. Similiarly, extended family is already prepared to provide assistance and may be more available and organized to help and provide support to parents.

The toddler (18-24 months) is beginning to exert independence and is learning to say no. Toddlers often exhibit aggressive, negative responses to treatment, which can make their care particularly exasperating and result in parents feeling guilty, apprehensive, and resentful.[6] These children experience separation from their mother more acutely than do younger babies and they are more likely to show marked changes in behavior during hospitalization. These changes may include temporary emotional withdrawal and loss of interest in the environment; diminished responsiveness; protest behavior with crying, fretfulness, temper outbursts, and extreme rebelliousness; or changes in sleeping, eating, and bowel habits. The toddler typically relinquishes recent accomplishments and returns to earlier patterns of feeding, toileting, thumb sucking, and language.

By early childhood (3-4 years), the child's strong dependent attachment to its mother is beginning to relax as the youngster strives for independence and becomes increasingly capable of managing much of his or her physical care. Sexual identity is developing, accompanied by feelings of love, rivalry, tenderness, and anger toward parents. The illness interferes with this growing independence and can produce demanding, irritable behavior.[6]

The child and family will concentrate on the various positive and negative effects of therapy once it has been started. Most chemotherapeutic drugs will take a toll on the child's appearance and general health. Hair loss often is the first and most dramatic change. Without adult interference, children under the age of 10 usually are not disturbed by baldness and often reject wigs, but preteen and adolescent patients whose developing self-image is still fragile and whose increasing independence from parents is complemented by strong kinship with peers usually are greatly distressed by becoming bald. The need for conformity peaks between the ages of 10 and 12, when expectations and judgments of group members can be harsh. Other conspicuous differences in appearance, such as excessive weight loss or gain, weakness, or disfigurement as a result of amputation or other invasive surgery, can also be devastating. In adolescence, the youngster is experimenting with many personae and beauty and physical strength and prowess are vital for status and self-esteem. To be unable to take one's body for granted, to feel vulnerable, and to lack physical well being produce extreme stress and sometimes anxiety. Even more than for younger children, the adolescent's self-identity is closely tied to acceptance by and belonging in a group. Adolescents cannot look to peers to help them with these concerns, nor can they be reassured by parents that friends will remain faithful and attentive.

Cancer separates adolescents from their peers in other ways as well. Awareness of his or her own mortality and the possibility of death and the exposure to the pain, sickness, and death of other young patients spurs growth beyond chronological age. The child must try to blend with friends who cannot share the illness and the personal experience in any meaningful way. Emotionally, adolescents suffer more than younger children. Although often they cannot think or feel beyond the present, they are also oriented to the future and are encouraged to think about careers and becoming independent from parents. Relationships can become turbulent as teenagers struggle for autonomy yet need to remain connected to family. Adolescents may avoid encounters with cancer peers until their therapy has been completed and they can feel that cancer is safely behind them. At this point, survivors look back on the illness, the period of treatment, and their parents' reactions from a secure vantage point.

Various side effects such as nausea and vomiting, mouth sores, muscle pain, and fatigue can result in varying amounts of time lost from school. Although most children are encouraged to continue attending, many miss a critical amount of schooling owing to actual or perceived medical problems. Intense regimens, low white cell counts, and the resulting risk of infection can mean isolation from peers and social life, thereby compromising the youngster's ability to reconnect. The chronically ill child typically relates better to adults than to peers and may be more thoughtful, less forthcoming, and more passive and emotional than other children of the same age.[9]

Young cancer patients must maintain a delicate balance between managing their body's response to the illness and their own emotions. As children grow, self-esteem is closely tied to self-care and self-control, both of which are taxed by the illness. Relationships with parents or with other caretakers are vital to a child who is seriously ill. Parents console and encourage their child. Their behavior and expectations tell the youngster much about his or her present and future. Parents' worries and fears are often adopted by the child; some youngsters attempt to nurture or protect their parents, probably as a way of helping themselves, because overwhelmed parents are not available as a source of comfort, which threatens the child's sense of security.

Younger children often tolerate the physical aspects of treatment better than older children. Because a young child is expected to be close to parents and may not verbalize fears and worries, psychological and social difficulties may not become manifest until later, when lack of socialization, missed schooling, parental overprotectiveness, and worry result in maladaptive behavior. Maladaptation may be exhibited by school phobias, psychosomatic symptoms which encourage school absence, inability to form and maintain friendships, lack of sensitivity to social cues, risk-taking and other self-destructive behavior, fears or night terrors, lack of emotional resilience, and misplaced anger. Although the best approach is prevention, parents often cannot respond to a social worker's interventions directed to circumvent future problems because concerns about the child's physical health take precedence. Many parents, however, are receptive to suggestions intended to enhance a child's present and future adjustment.

A child who has successfully adjusted to the illness has had to contend with an array of pressures and frustrations. Perhaps a critical stage of growth has been disrupted but he or she has been able to reconnect with important developmental tasks, maintain trust in significant adults, and develop a secure self-identity. Maturity brings increased intellectual understanding, variety in modes of expression, and improved judgment, all assets that help the child contend with adversity. Acquaintance and association with others who have been successful in managing similar problems can support development of a positive self-image. Many youngsters display pride and confidence in themselves as they successfully master the ongoing stress associated with their illness.[10]

STAFF AND INSTITUTIONAL FACTORS

The onset of cancer in a pediatric patient constitutes a major crossroads in which hospital caregivers and family members connect in encounters that are heightened by emotional intensity. The diagnosis exposes the vulnerability of children and adults; magnifies the already awesome responsibility of the medical professionals; and heralds enormous, irreversible, and often unforeseeable changes in the family. Health professionals become intimate partners with individuals, heretofore strangers, whose lives become greatly influenced by these relationships and by actions taken on their behalf. Staff, in turn, are profoundly affected by patients and family members, by the extent of their responsibility, and by the meaning and importance of their mission. A family's fragile adaptive mechanisms early in the childhood cancer experience can be thwarted or hindered by negative, confusing, or unproductive interactions with staff and by institutional procedures or circumstances.

When parents are trying to grasp what is happening to their child and the intricacies of proposed therapy, the manner and amount of information presented to them may be pivotal. Parents do not have the luxury of time to react to the diagnosis and to recover sufficiently from the shock to ask questions before making decisions about treatment.

In the current health care system that uses diagnostic related groupings (DRGs) and minimized inpatient hospital stays, children with cancer may not be permitted enough inpatient days for the parents to have adjusted sufficiently before they are taking home a child with a life-threatening illness. The timing of discharge usually is dictated by the child's medical condition, but a family's preparedness to accept the child at home is based on other factors. So much information must be presented that parents are literally talking or being talked to much of the time. Vital information may be provided by skilled attending clinicians, less-experienced fellows, residents, or interns recently out of medical school. All professionals have personal feelings, philosophies, self-expectations, experiences, and a need for appreciation or admiration that can influence how information is presented. A team approach is ideal because social workers and nurses can contribute, soften, or stimulate further explanation of medical facts. However, many people will interact with the family, posing the risk that the parents will become confused, fearful, or angry.

Parents cannot, of course, be guaranteed a cure for their child and even those patients whose diseases are considered eminently treatable are at risk for a relapse and eventual death from cancer, infection, or another complication. If the words "fatal" or "death" are never mentioned in connection with their child's illness, parents cannot form realistic expectations and their adjustment will be more difficult, especially if things do not proceed smoothly.

All parents seek a positive outcome and even when given little assurance can find a spark of hope. Sometimes parents will ask for (or doctors will freely offer) statistics regarding length of survival and outcome; but statistics do not tell them what will happen to *their* child or help them prepare for the future.

Even as parents are told that here is no guaranteed cure, they should be told that the disease can be treated, that their child will likely be discharged from the hospital, and that he or she can lead a normal life in spite of the need for continued treatment and surveillance. As communicators, social workers concentrate on what the physician tells the parents and the patient and the way it is being received by them. The social worker can help the doctor to accept that the truth will help, not harm the family. In family meetings the social worker can obtain a relevant history and elicit information about previous experiences, attitudes, and misconceptions to assure that information is presented to the family in language or within a context that has relevance to their particular situation or experience. By interacting with family members following medically focused meetings, the social worker can restate, interpret, and clarify information; help formulate, frame, or raise questions; and identify the need for additional meetings and arrange them. With the parents, the social worker can sort throughout the sometimes conflicting statements made by various medical personnel and encourage the parents to consider how the medical plan will affect their family.

Although many err by being excessively optimistic, some doctors may paint such a bleak outcome or describe unpleasant side effects in such graphic detail that the family refuses therapy that would prolong life, offer palliation, or have the potential to cure. The parents should be made aware that although few children may have been "cured" many have lived lives of good quality, and they should be apprised of instances of long-term survival or cure of their child's particular illness. Parents who have had personal experiences with or knowledge of adults who have cancer may view treatment as torture. Unless they are informed, they cannot know that treatment also palliates and that the experience of untreated cancer can be worse than enduring the side effects of cancer therapy.

Words used to describe to the patient and family the toxicity or discomfort of medical procedures should be chosen carefully but realistically. All professionals who work with cancer families know a great deal more than the parents or patient can know about what the future holds. Caregivers may become accustomed to or shield themselves from the unpleasant, even gruesome side effects of therapy. On the other hand, medical personnel cannot deliver to the family their own worst fears or withhold from them completely the possibility of adverse reactions. This is the crux of informed consent, that parents and the patient will benefit from explanations that encourage them to prepare realistically. The child, especially, will benefit because children's fears are specific to detail and their imaginations can lead them to unrealistic fears.

In pediatric oncology, length of survival is usually measured in years. Efforts to improve survival for patients who have diseases with less favorable prognoses have resulted in stratified treatment regimens, some of which are associated with much greater morbidity than others. Most centers, however, are dedicated to maintaining the quality of the child's life. Awareness of this concern, and of the fact that the therapy is adjusted to the patient's level of tolerance, is reassuring to parents, especially during the diagnostic and treatment induction phases of the illness.

American consumers of medicine are encouraged to ask questions and to seek the best care available. Gone are the days when doctors' prescriptions were automatically accepted without question. In the current environment of medical practice, caregivers are sometimes thrust into adversarial relationships with consumers. A multidisciplinary approach can prevent or ease conflicts. Social workers can assist with perceptions that members of the team have about assertive, questioning, untrusting families and also can help family members to understand how medical protocols are designed and how decisions are made for care and treatment. Such efforts are vital to helping build and maintain the trust that must exist when a child is diagnosed with cancer.

American society is influenced by a no-time-to-wait mentality. People have come to expect immediate service and immediate answers to difficult questions. Medical institutions do not work in this fashion. Rules and regulations and institutional arrangements, created ultimately for efficient diagnosis and treatment, can be perceived as dehumanizing and unbending. Although staff can help to soften the way parents perceive restrictions, parents may focus on issues that seem peripheral such as lack of cleanliness of a patient's room, the time medications are administered, or waiting for admission to the hospital, because they need someone or something upon which to discharge anger. When such complaints are justified, however, staff may need to acknowledge the legitimacy of such anger. It is not productive for parents to display or to feel anger towards persons in whose care they have entrusted their child. Moreover, exerting control over some aspect of the illness experience can be helpful at a time when there can be little control.

Difficulties of treatment, and the costs to the family, should not be downplayed. Parents must rearrange their lives, meet needs of their other children, and become partners in the care of the patient. Management of a child with cancer is so complex yet so compartmentalized that even physicians may not understand the issues and difficulties involved in care at home.

Honoring generational boundaries is an important component of helping families cope. The trend to provide consumers with total information at times extends inappropriately to the child. Parents are urged to provide their child facts about the illness and how it will be treated. This will communicate to the child that cancer is something he or she will be able to deal with, because children know that they are usually protected from things they cannot handle. However, information should be presented to the parents and the child (including the adolescent) separately, as the context and the words used for each will be different. Parents need an opportunity to recover and then consider what and how to tell their child. Social workers rarely are knowledgeable about a particular family prior to the diagnostic meeting and cannot predict how they will react when they are told about their child's illness. A young patient's exposure to an excessive display of parental emotions, vulnerability, and fear should be minimized, if possible. The parents need time to regain their composure, to share with their child feelings of sadness about the illness and the hospitalization, and to express hope to the child that the treatment will lead to recovery.

Development of positive relationships with staff is an important coping skill. Parents depend on and must give to others great responsibility for their child and the way that staff members interact with the family can encourage or discourage trust. The parents have a right to expect that, although they must relinquish their child to professionals for treatment of the disease, they are still in charge of their child and retain control over other aspects of the child's life. While parents can benefit from experience, suggestions, and guidance, social workers' actions should not disrupt generational boundaries or lose perspective of the fact that the patient is the parents' child.

SOCIOECONOMIC IMPLICATIONS

Treatment of pediatric cancer is a complex combination of inpatient and outpatient care that requires parents of a child with cancer to deal with numerous billing offices.[11] Negotiation of this system requires knowledge and fortitude.

Some families will perceive a medical catastrophe in terms of its fiscal dimensions. By focusing thoughts and emotions on practical and financial details, parents can ease the anxiety they feel about whether their child will live or die. Requests for information regarding the financial aspects of the illness may offer an outlet for attending to *something* in an unhappy, uncertain atmosphere. Complaints about hospital accounting procedures or parking rates can serve as vehicles for releasing anger. The impact of the illness and related practical and affective tasks can drain the parents to the point that they have few emotional and practical reserves available for coping with medical charges, insurance claims, and other details of payment. In comparison to cancer, bills, other children, employment, and household chores may seem insignificant.

The medical bill may symbolize past or future medical care provided to the child: If it is paid, the child will fare well; if the child dies, perhaps the parents aren't obligated to pay the hospital or the doctors. Such ways of thinking about or using money are aspects of *bargaining*, a common behavioral expression of the parents' desire to take control over or to influence the course of the illness. Especially during the first year after the diagnosis, families may bestow personal gifts or donations to a favorite cause or charity. Gift giving becomes a way of saying "thank you" and of assuring that nothing is overlooked in the effort to save their child.

A family's socioeconomic history will influence its members' capacity to withstand financial strain, their attitudes towards the expenses associated with the illness, and their ability to budget and seek new resources. Economic problems can hamper a family's ability to conform to the treatment routine, manage emotional stress, and maintain a family life.

For the very poor, the illness may diminish in importance in proportion to the ongoing struggle to provide for basic necessities. Decisions regarding treatment either for cure or palliation may be influenced by the crisis of the day. Extreme poverty often is compounded by other social and health problems such as family disorganization, poor education, school maladjustment, domestic violence, or substance abuse. With the disease, the need for goods and services is intensified.[11]

Families confronted with a child who has cancer face daunting tasks: Obtain information about the anticipated costs of the child's illness, asses family requirements and available funds, reorder priorities, adjust budgets, and perhaps learn to budget for the first time. The parents must also procure new resources, a task influenced by the ability to realistically appraise financial circumstances and a willingness to disclose facts about family income and holdings. By necessity, a family's self-image as an independent, self-sufficient unit must change. A need for financial help represents a blow to personal pride and families will have different ways of dealing with it. Some may feel that accepting money from extended family or friends is less objectionable than accepting funds from public or private charities; others may avoid asking relatives for help because doing so could intensify or revive past or present conflicts. In other instances, material assistance may be freely offered but rejected because it is seen as a substitute for emotional support or personal involvement in the family's plight. Social workers can learn much about a family by asking a number of pertinent questions about its use of money. Answers to questions about who earns the family income or who decides how money is spent can reveal as much about relationships and balances of power as about household economics.

A child's cancer challenges accustomed and comfortable role assignments. In traditional families, the father earns the money and influences how it is spent, while the mother tends to children and the home.What if the mother cannot fulfill expected duties because she is needed at the hospital? Will the father assume some of the child care and household duties? Whether he takes on "domestic" tasks, his status at home, with friends, and at work may be affected. Will the father resent having to go to work and feel excluded from the events at the hospital?

Today, however, it is common for both parents to be employed and it may be impractical or unacceptable for the mother to stay home with the ill child. A mother's career and her paycheck may be essential to fulfillment of family goals, the income may be crucial to meeting mortgage or other financial obligations, or her employer may be the source of the health insurance that pays for the patient's medical care. Mother's role as breadwinner may influence her decision-making power in other areas of family life including decisions about the patient's medical care.

Authority regarding how a family's income is used may be shared or considered the prerogative of only one partner. These arrangements may be disrupted by the child's illness. Changes in roles or authority affect decisions about how financial resources are expended. Unwillingness to form new family or personal goals and priorities can result in unrealistic spending in the face of increasing financial burdens.

A family overwhelmed by debts can be strained to the breaking point. Families who can be flexible about roles can accommodate adjustment of schedules, duties, and expectations and maintain financial and emotional stability and grow stronger as a family.

Divorced, reconstituted, and single-parent families face particular challenges that may rekindle old disputes and threaten newly formed families. Often, contact between estranged spouses is spurred by a need to work out financial arrangements or to renew claims to the child.

An unmarried or widowed parent who must work faces a tremendous struggle in striving to provide care for a seriously ill or dying child. The single parent is locked into the role of breadwinner and primary caretaker and is exceptionally vulnerable. In some instances independence is forfeited as grandparents' aid in caring for the sick child is elicited.

BEYOND THE DIAGNOSTIC PHASE

The phases past the period of diagnosis are remission, relapse, terminal illness and bereavement, and long-term survival and begin with the child's discharge from the hospital. At each point in the disease process, whether it culminates in the child's cure or the child's death, the family must be guided in its search for ways to cope and adjust.

RETURNING HOME

Until recently, the first hospitalization of a child with newly diagnosed malignancy was extended until the child had adjusted, and perhaps responded, to an initial course of treatment. The hospital stay was generally long enough for relationships to be formed between staff and family. This scenario today is the exception rather than the rule and often the new patient is discharged before anyone in the family has had sufficient time to grasp basic facts about the disease and the treatment. Parents still reeling from the diagnosis and the first hospitalization are expected to deliver highly technical care at home with a brief period of training. In the past, parents experienced relief at discharge because going home was an indication that the child was doing well. Now, with intermittent assistance from visiting nurses, parents are assuming home care of children whose condition may be barely stable.

One of the difficulties of these trends is that health professionals are not afforded an opportunity to get to know the family, except superficially, and often only tentative relationships can be developed. Therefore, the ability to anticipate or circumvent families' problems is diminished. At the same time, medical care now is more complicated and more fragmented and even educated parents may be so overcome emotionally that they cannot absorb or properly integrate information. Thrust into roles once carried out by health care professionals in a hospital, at home they may become confused or not respond to signs indicative of infection or respiratory distress. Or, parents may not trust themselves at all and bring the child back to the hospital for minor or imagined problems.

Single-parent families, families that are disorganized, or families who have little or no extended family support can be strained to the breaking point if expectations for home care are not compatible with their resources. Social workers are crucial to successful discharge planning because they are trained to make appropriate and necessary assessments of the family's ability to manage at home.

Parents generally are apprehensive about the first discharge from the hospital because they are taking home a different child–one who has cancer and who might die. The parents may be unsure of how to behave toward this child and of what to expect of him or her. If a child acts out rebelliously because of overexposure to parents' distress or uncertainty, a vicious cycle maybe set in motion. Behavior becomes more unmanageable in response to parental insecurity about discipline, and feelings of guilt prevent parents from exerting control over the child's unacceptable conduct.

REMISSION

Once the home care routine is established, most families usually move away from a crisis mode and regain equilibrium. If the child is in remission and the disease has responded to the treatment, then hope for a positive outcome is strengthened. Remission means, in some cases, that no cancer can be detected; in other cases, remission means that the disease progression has been arrested. Of course, as with the initial diagnostic period, the quality of this time depends on many factors. The prognosis, toleration of treatment, side effects experienced, the social and emotional responses of family, friends and the community, all contribute to the family's adjustment during the remission phase.

If the child feels well and can return to normal activities and if the demands of treatment are not too great, then the parents may be able to de-emphasize the child as a patient.[4] This is a healthy response and should be encouraged. Many parents, however, will find it difficult to treat the child as before because of restrictions imposed by the medical regimen, the child's diminished strength, or because of fears about the child's safety. Parents may have difficulty achieving an appropriate balance of protective behavior and encouraging independence without supportive counseling.

Although certain protocols require periodic rehospitalization, most children receive outpatient care. The trend toward giving chemotherapy and antibiotics at home is likely to increase. Adjustment to the outpatient clinic setting is difficult for some parents who are accustomed to more individualized medical attention and feel uncomfortable with the public, open quality that characterizes most outpatient programs. Further, long waiting periods and exposure to other very ill children can be stressful.

In some instances, parents who have apparently coped very well during the diagnostic period experience difficulty in the remission period. The parent who temporarily "collapses" after the crisis has subsided may have waited until it was "safe" to do so. Also, it appears that some parents actively regulate their grieving.[12]

Eventually the family joins the oncology "system," in which having a child with cancer is the norm.[5] Outside of the hospital system, being parents of a cancer patient sets them apart. They may not feel comfortable discussing the child's illness and treatment with friends, relatives, coworkers, or teachers at the school where the patient or siblings are enrolled. All family members struggle to remain connected with former friends and pastimes, despite the reality that they are irrevocably changed. The hospital and staff can come to feel as close as home and family.

With the passage of time, the sense of crisis diminishes and other family problems may re-emerge or develop. There now may be energy to invest in a treatment relationship. During these periods, developmental issues can receive attention as the child is seen as having a life and therefore a future. School attendance and performance and social relationships can now be considered.

Indicators of maladaptive parental coping during remission are prolonged focus on death, excessive worry, resisting the patient's return to school, isolating the child from peers, and abandonment of orthodox treatment in favor of quack or unorthodox ones.[4]

Schooling Issues

The cancer patient's re-entry to school may take place after a brief or a prolonged period of absence. Depending on how the child is changed as a result of the illness, the child's adjustment maybe difficult or smooth. The role of the hospital teacher can be helpful in facilitating the child's adjustment. Reduced vitality may restrict attendance to only a portion of the day or week and may interfere with participation in usual activities. Certain cancers affect the child's ability to function in the usual classroom setting. With brain tumors, for example, the child may have blurred vision, coordination difficulties, or other impediments that make writing or reading difficult. On the other hand, many youngsters can fully participate in school and should be encouraged to attend. Even marginal attendance, supplemented with home tutoring, is preferable to total nonattendance. Children can catch up with missed academic work more readily than they can regain lost social contacts. Ongoing social and emotional development is contingent upon involvement with other children in normal settings and cannot be simulated in the home environment.

As a result of certain treatments, primarily irradiation to the central nervous system, some cancer patients will suffer minimal to severe brain damage that will affect learning and school performance. These deficits are not always predictable nor do they follow a clear-cut pattern, but they may involve memory loss, sequencing difficulties, inattentiveness, and trouble concentrating. In some cases, children have lost as many as 30 points on IQ tests.[13] Since the discovery of this problem patients have been treated with lower doses of radiation, but it is still too soon to know whether these adverse late effects will be avoided.[13] Social problems such as immaturity, lack of judgment, and absence of ambition and passivity have also been noted, particularly in children who have received therapy for brain tumors. The way the family responds to these social, emotional, and physical deficits can hinder or assist the child's adjustment.

Many treatment centers offer individualized help with educational problems and techniques have been developed to assist teachers in handling the particular learning problems of these children. But other factors can influence the youngster's successful integration into school. Because of a cancer patient's physical appearance or the life-threatening nature of the illness, teachers may be uncomfortable interacting with the patient or parents and attempt to protect themselves from establishing emotional contact with these students. The obvious association of cancer with death may lead a teacher to assume that the child will become critically ill while at school or cannot participate in activities even though the child may be feeling well and optimistic about the future.[14] Programs that help educate teachers can prove very useful in these situations.[15]

RELAPSE

The prognosis for any particular form of cancer depends largely upon the current level of scientific knowledge. Although therapies are available against virtually every type of childhood cancer, the lack of a specific cure means that in many cases the disease will recur. The first remission usually is the longest and with few exceptions relapse generally means that the child will not survive. The family again faces uncertainty because it is impossible to predict how the disease will respond to new therapies. Many children live for years after a relapse, but others die only months or weeks after relapse. The availability of effective therapies is an important factor: Death is inevitable if there is no way to treat the disease.

Some cancers are extremely virulent and aggressive and either do not respond to therapy or recur after brief or unstable periods of remission. Other types respond to an array of therapies and the patient may live many years despite multiple relapses. As during the diagnosis phase, the nature of the disease and the child's response will affect the way a family deals with relapse. If the remission period has been long and uneventful, with infrequent visits to the clinic the only reminders of cancer, the seriousness of the illness may have become a fading memory, with cure an attained goal. Relapse is especially devastating for families with such high hopes because it is unexpected. If the patient has had a very difficult course, the full significance of relapse may not be obvious. Interpretation of the meaning of relapse should always include a realistic appraisal of the changed prognosis and expectations for the quality of survival. The family whose hopes are diminished must face the probability of death yet remain connected to the child, who more than ever needs their love, support, and attention.[4]

In some instances, as in testicular relapse in leukemia, the relapse does not necessarily predict a negative outcome. With some cancers, bone marrow transplants offer the chance for potentially curative therapies to be administered. However, the consideration of research treatment, as well as of marrow transplants, carries with it a host of issues that have a profound impact on the family.

Regardless of whether further treatment may be possible, parents who respond to the news of relapse by withdrawing from their child need to be encouraged to maintain hope and treat their child as if he or she has a life. Whether or not death is anticipated, distancing from a youngster who is alert and interacting with others is dysfunctional. Parents may need help to rekindle hope; if cure is not possible, perhaps for some other cherished goal.

Relapse reactivates the crisis, as parents and other family members anticipate the loss of the child. Families who adapted poorly during the initial phase of the illness will have problems adjusting when the cancer recurs. The effects of maladaptation may be cumulative; the family could experience relapse as if the diagnosis were never known.[4] Starting over with a new round of treatment and side effects and less hope for the future is difficult. The youngster is likely to be more aware of the demands of cancer therapy as well as the possibility of death.[4] Parental feelings of relatedness to the child have intensified or diminished as a result of the illness. Relapse may reactivate clinging or further withdrawal; both can be emotionally disruptive for the child and the other members of the family.

Patients and families who cope effectively with a relapse include those who are knowledgeable about the illness and who have benefitted from relationships with children who died and their families. The experiences of others suggest to the child and family a course of events that can be anticipated and rehearsed emotionally.[4]

TERMINAL PERIOD

When conventional therapy is no longer effective in controlling a child's malignancy, parents must make decisions regarding continuation of treatment with investigational drugs or initiation of palliative care. There are considerable variations regarding how patient and family should be apprised at this significant juncture. Treatment centers may not have standardized decision-making processes for continued aggressive therapy. Interpretation of options is the responsibility of the physician, whose point of view will be prominent, but whether there is a no-holds-barred approach to last-ditch efforts or gentle guidance toward cessation of therapy and preparation for the child's death, other members of the health care team and, most importantly, the family and child, should participate in decision making. This is a time of ambivalence. Parents may be able to grasp intellectually that death is inevitable, yet may be unable emotionally to accept or believe that their child will die.[4]

Although some families and physicians desire to battle for the child's life to the end and interpret discontinuance of treatment as a betrayal of the child, caregivers and parents often can acknowledge the inevitable and shift priorities from cure to palliation. The terminal phase is an anguished but crucial period that affords everyone involved an opportunity to talk about death, to raise questions, and to make plans. It is the beginning of a process of memorializing the child that will continue years after the death. Families with a closed style of communication cannot be expected to convert suddenly to an open and expressive style, but during times of crisis families often are willing to consider alternative behaviors and to receive assistance as they come to grips with the impending death of their child. The terminal period in the child's illness helps family members accomplish several important tasks: *rehearsal,* which involves realistic preparation of practical and emotional aspects of the death; *letting go,* in which they begin to accept death and loosen ties to the loved one; *grief work,* in which they experience the pain associated with loss; and *memorialization,* in which they select and refine positive thoughts and memories.

One important consideration is deciding *where* the child will die. Despite the influence of hospice care, most persons have been shielded from the experience of death. Memories of the final days of family members and friends often involve hospital rooms, machines, and tubes. Even though active medical treatment has been discontinued and supportive care initiated, the terminally ill child may feel well and not be in need of hospitalization.[8] Children focus on the present and need no urging to take advantage of a good day or hour. Home care for the children often is not complex and the family will be less disrupted if the dying child is cared for at home.[8] Family participation in the care of a child dying at home may reduce the feelings of hopelessness, anxiety, stress, and guilt. A reduction in the intensity of these feelings may alter or expedite the resolution of grief after a child's death.[16]

Home care allows parents and siblings to intimately and informally interact with the patient. Emotional preparation for death may be expedited by the consideration of the many details surrounding the event that serves as a kind of rehearsal, and by the minute changes observed in the child's condition that herald the approaching death. The home can become a source of unpleasant memories as the place where the child died, however, and social workers may need to help the survivors dissipate these references so that normal family life can resume.[8] In some instances, family preferences and needs may dictate that hospitalization during terminal care is a better arrangement.

Parents whose child is active and actively relating to them may have difficulty focusing on death, yet it is important that they be engaged in planning to meet the needs of this *living* child. Decisions regarding activities, education, visits from friends, and sharing of information with the child are important. A child who feels well will appreciate being active and busy. It is not unusual at this time for patients to attend school or receive home tutoring because school is an integral and valued part of a child's life and offers connections with friends and accomplishments. Classmates and educators will benefit from the social worker's help with questions that arise and emotions that are evoked. Eventually, increased fatigue, emotional withdrawal, and other signs of approaching death will limit activities.

Although some parents can discuss the subject of death openly, most parents recoil from talking with their child about death. Children's ideas, fears, and questions about death vary considerably, as does their ability to verbalize them. Parents' attitudes and the child's experience with death will determine what is imagined and said. It is not uncommon for children to withhold thoughts and ideas they perceive will distress their parents. The child should not be left to deal alone with fears and worries. Although parents are the right persons to address these concerns, they may need help in managing their feelings and finding the best words to use with their child. There is a context within each family to discuss questions about death in a way that can be comforting to the patient. The social worker can help the parents verbalize what they believe are their child's concerns and rehearse appropriate responses.Most children experience death anxiety as fear of abandonment or of separation from parents and parents can provide reassurance that they will not leave the child.[4]

Siblings should be prepared for the death and be told that efforts to make the child well will continue. They should never be given the impression that doctors or the family have given up on a brother or sister. Often siblings display symptoms that mimic those experienced by the patient because they perceive illness as a means of obtaining attention from parents.[8]

The death of a sibling precipitates an emotional crisis with a far-reaching and pervasive impact. The meaning of the death depends upon many factors, including the particular developmental stage of the sibling and his or her ability to conceptualize the finality and irreversibility of death. Natural rivalry between siblings and resentment because of parents' exclusive focus on the sick child can lead to a wish for the death of the one who has received coveted emotional and material attention. However, some children feel responsible for a sick brother or sister and blame themselves for failing to protect their sibling.[8] Siblings may experience isolation in the aftermath of the death of a brother or sister. Conflicted and unexpressed feelings, limited understanding of the event, or observations of the profound and tragic nature of parental grief and the parents' need for privacy create a kind of shield between parents and surviving children. A child may not also be able to confide in parents because the child fears the parents' disapproval or anger but also because lack of life experience and immaturity make it difficult to verbalize such feelings.[8]

The loss of a sister or brother profoundly affects the fragile, developing sense of self which is intimately connected with family and the unique place the child occupies within it. The meaning of a sibling's death will change, gaining or losing prominence as time passes and the survivor moves through various life stages.

Siblings who are at least 4 years old should be involved in decisions regarding attendance at the funeral. At this age, a child can be given a clear picture of what to expect, including the outpouring of emotions, and on the basis of this information can be helped to make a decision to attend a portion of the funeral events. A bereaved brother or sister must never be forced to participate in the funeral. Those who do attend need support and direction from adults and should not be left alone.

BEREAVEMENT

Parental bereavement differs from other types of bereavement in intensity and duration. A child's death induces a profound sense of failure. This aspect adds another dimension to the experience of loss and can threaten self-confidence and feelings of self-worth. Both parents grieve and difficulty in supporting one another is a consequence. Therefore, the most natural therapeutic resource for each is unavailable. Parental grief may continue longer and intensify more frequently because parents demarcate their lives by events in the lives of their children, alive or dead.[17]

Although social workers recognize the loss of any child as unnatural and a tragedy, certain deaths can be more difficult for parents. A death that is sudden and unexpected does not give parents time to cherish the child in the special way evoked by the anticipated loss and robs parents of the opportunity to participate in activities that may thwart or forestall death. In most cases of childhood cancer, there is a period of disease remission during which parents are helped to prepare for the loss through passage of time, acceptance of the seriousness of the illness, management of adverse side effects, and awareness of other children who die. Parents know what their child has undergone, can see and sense the subtle and obvious changes. So that, after a time of fighting disease, if the child becomes more ill and is unable to enjoy previous pleasures and withdraws from activities and friends, there is a kind of reasonableness attached to the death. Death brings an end to suffering and struggle. Parents can take comfort in knowing they had done everything possible to help their child and that their love was demonstrated.

The mourning process is not completely understood, but it is known that there are various stages, each with a different focus and character. Usually there is a period of numbness, a time of emotional anesthesia that enables parents to organize and participate in practical tasks. After some weeks, the numbness subsides and more intense feelings of pain and loss are experienced. Eventually, parents feel despair as they realize that their child will never return. The timing of these stages is unfortunate because friends and family usually are the most solicitous in the days and weeks immediately following a death. It is not unusual for these associates to withdraw or not be available to discuss the deceased child or aspects of the illness and death. Finally, there is a time of reorganization and renewal as ties to the lost child have been loosened and the bereaved recover. It may take many years for a parent to reach this stage.

Some parents seem to regulate the emotional intensity of their responses, which results in a postponement of mourning. The onset of delayed grief is unexpected and may immobilize persons who previously functioned well. Other problems during bereavement occur when parents do not allow themselves to heal and inflict or accentuate pain by reliving unhappy memories. Self-inflicted pain is a way to revive the most intense emotions connected to the child, but it is not a healthy response to the loss and may be an indicator of serious pathology.

As with the illness, parents' way of coping with death and its aftermath and their expectations of one another may not match. One parent may be expressive while the other parent has a need to control emotions, or as a way of protecting a partner, feelings are concealed. Somatic complaints, commonly associated with grief, can prevent participation in familiar activities or inhibit sexual relations. The resulting dissynchrony can disrupt communication and threaten the marital relationship.

Problems in the family that had low priority during the illness may resurface and complicate or confuse the grief process. Disheartened parents may be unable to devote themselves to working on other issues and other losses intensify feelings of vulnerability. The world becomes a dangerous place in which children get cancer and die.

Religious beliefs, which ascribe meaning to the loss, may serve as compensation for bereaved parents. Such beliefs include expectations for reunion with the deceased child in Heaven and explanations for the death in terms of a higher, noble purpose.[18] Parents who view their child's death as punishment for wrongdoing may have no compensation. Such attitudes are usually pre-existent and may be observed throughout the illness.

Months after a child's death, it is common for parents to have many questions regarding the efficacy of various medical interventions. These questions arise as the parents attempt to organize and integrate the illness and its aftermath into their self and world concepts. Unless an autopsy had been performed, it may be impossible to provide answers to their questions. Discussions about autopsy prior to or at the time of a child's death should explain the procedure as one that provides answers to parents' as well as caregivers' questions. These answers can help the patient's family as well as other children with the same disease.

ENDING THERAPY

If a remission has been unbroken or regained and the course of treatment has been completed (a period that may last a few months or three years), the child is taken off therapy. This is an important hallmark for parents and the patient and often is celebrated with parties, gifts, and general rejoicing. While coming off treatment is symbolic of cure, it does not guarantee that the cancer will not return. At this juncture some parents and patients experience a letdown; although the therapy was abhorred, it was a part of being actively treated. Without therapy the child seems unprotected and concerns about relapse may arise. At the point where cure seems more than an uncertain hope, the family and patient feel a renewed sense of vulnerability.

An older child who appears elated when treatment is successfully completed later may exhibit diminished self-confidence, periods of overwhelming sadness, absence of motivation, and inability to concentrate, all reminiscent of grief reactions or the despondence which often follows acute episodes of illness. These responses are normal sequelae of a long ordeal, but assistance with reordering the experience can help the former patient fit the illness more comfortably into the rest of his or her life.[19]

As time off treatment lengthens, former patients may become more aware and less accepting of the permanent physical changes or deficits that resulted from the cancer or its treatment. The young adult, struggling to find a place in life, may express strong resentment and blame parents for what has been done.[19] Even relatively minor deficits can be a source of discomfort and emotional pain to a young man or woman who does not want to be different from peers.

Survivorship may also bring maturity beyond chronical age because of what has been endured and the uncomfortable awareness of personal mortality. Often more serious-minded than healthy peers, survivors may feel isolated and distant from them. If motivated to make new friends and to form new goals and aspirations more in keeping with the persons they have become, cancer survivors may attain a better sense of self. Other survivors compensate for feelings of inferiority and dependency with high-risk-taking behavior.[20] Decreased self-esteem and a pervasive sense of mutability can inhibit investment in interpersonal relationships and a career.[18]

The persistent sense of vulnerability that results from having escaped a potential death sentence can make it difficult for survivors of childhood cancer to endure minor physical complaints such as viral infections. Excessive worry and fear triggered by vivid memories of past problems are easily evoked and admission to a hospital, even for surgery to ameliorate minor functional or cosmetic defects, is distressing.[19] A younger child may not remember details or actual events but will recall painful apprehensions of the past experience when returning to the hospital.

Parents who have been vigilant and protective of their child during the course of treatment may find it difficult to step back and allow the child to be more independent. Parents who eagerly awaited the freedom afforded by the child's continued health and maturity may need to adjust their hopes and expectations if intellectual, emotional, or physical problems limit their child's achievement of complete independence.[19]

Tasks that require a former childhood cancer patient to recall the past, such as completing a job application or preparing a biographical statement as part of admission to a university, may trigger feelings of discomfort. The young adult who was treated during childhood may have only vague and selective recollections of that time. Parents who wish their son or daughter to keep the disease in the past or who are loathe to relive their own painful memories may discourage discussion of the experience. The person may feel that harboring such a dangerous or burdensome secret does not give them the freedom to divulge facts about the illness for the fear of losing status or employment.[19]

ETHICAL ISSUES FOR THE SOCIAL WORKER [21]

Value issues are commonly addressed in medical settings, and particularly when a specific cure for a disease being treated does not exist. In pediatric cancer, these ethical issues arise from many factors: The uncertainty of outcome; the manipulation of children who cannot make decisions for themselves; the difficulty of obtaining informed consent because of the complex nature of the disease and treatment; the intense long-term involvement of patient and family with medical staffs and treatment centers; the sometimes conflicting interests of researcher, healer, parent and patient; and the varying roles and expectations of many caregivers.[21] Social workers' many roles–family counselor, advocate, colleague, and nonmedical staff person–create distinctive value conflicts that must be resolved so that families can receive the best care.

Pediatric oncology social workers help parents make difficult choices regarding the treatment of their child and often participate with medical staff in making decisions that can have extensive and long-range influence on the family and patient. Confidentiality and other constraints imposed by the social work profession must be respected; social workers must make their assessment of and interpret to others family situations or points of view in ways that do not violate trust. Social workers also have obligations to children, who have the right to receive treatments that may cure, prolong life, or offer palliation. Client-related issues must be balanced with institutional goals and in the midst of these complex situations social workers must make ethical decisions. Social workers in pediatric oncology are obliged to stretch their ethical capacity and continue to develop.[22]

CONCLUSION

The family of a child diagnosed with cancer has a tremendous burden thrust upon it. Each phase of the illness requires that family members cope with new circumstances dictated by a disease in which the only predictable course is uncertainty about the patient's future.

The family of a child who has cancer is a family in need, regardless of the emotional or financial resources available to its members.

Social workers bring a particular combination of skills and training to the multidisciplinary pediatric cancer-care team. This expertise enables social workers to assess parents' strengths and weaknesses, ability to cope, communication styles, value systems, and a myriad of other factors that come into play during a time crisis. Possessed of such knowledge, social workers can then formulate and carry out plans of care that will help meet a family's needs.

The intense emotions felt and expressed in response to a cancer diagnosis are amplified if the new cancer patient is a child. From this vantage point, the social worker has a pivotal role as care of the family becomes a component in the care of the child. Some parents may require only minimal help in adjusting their lives. Some families may have needs so great that social workers skills and professional resources are taxed. Regardless of the interventions required, families of children with cancer will benefit from social workers' contributions to the caregiving team.

Advances in cancer treatment and care have contributed to a new aspect of the oncology social worker's practice–the aspect of survivorship. While sickness and death will be the unfortunate total of some families' experiences with childhood cancer, effective therapies mean that some pediatric cancers are curable. Increasingly, children who survived the disease and the rigors of treatment are going on to lead cancer-free lives. In this respect, although the social worker's task in caring for a young patients' family may have a beginning, it may not have a clearly demarcated end. Long-term survivorship is a positive outcome of a cancer diagnosis and the social worker is uniquely positioned to address the issues associated with it.

REFERENCES

1. Futterman EH, Hoffman I. Crisis and adaptation in the families of fatally ill children. In: Anthony J, Koupernick C, eds. *The Child in His Family, the Impact of Disease and Death, vol. 2.* New York, NY: John Wiley & Sons; 1973.

2. Moos RH, Tsu VD. The crisis of physical illness: an overview. In: Moos RH, ed. *Coping with Physical Illness.* New York, NY: Plenum Medical Book Company; 1979: 3-21.

3. Caroff P, Mailick M. The patient has a family: reaffirming social work's domain. *Social Work in Health Care.* 1985;10:17-34.

4. Ross JW. Social work intervention with families of children with cancer: the changing critical phases. *Social Work in Health Care.* 1978;3:257-272.

5. Ross JW. Coping with childhood cancer: group intervention as an aid to parents in crisis. *Social Work in Health Care.* 1979; 4:381-391.

6. McCollom AT. Coping with prolonged health impairment. In: *Your Child.* Boston, Mass: Little Brown & Co; 1975.

7. Ross JW, Klar H. Mental health practice in a physical health setting. *Social Casework.* 1982; March:147-154.

8. Ross JW. Hospice care for children: psychosocial considerations. In: *Quality of Care for theTerminally Ill: An Examination of Issues.* A special publication of the *Quality Review Bulletin*, Joint Commission on Accreditation of Hospitals, Chicago, Ill: 1985;124-131.

9. Spinetta JJ, Deasy-Spinetta P, eds. *Living with Childhood Cancer.* St. Louis, Mo: CV Mosby; 1981.

10. Mattson A. Long-term physical illness in childhood: a challenge to psychosocial adaptation. *Pediatrics.* 1972;50:801-811.

11. Bonnem S, Ross JW. Financial issues in pediatric cancer. In: Pizzo PA, Poplack DG, eds. *Principles and Practice of Pediatric Oncology.* Philadelphia, Pa: JB Lippincott Co; 1988;915-922.

12. Futterman EH, Hoffman I, Sabshin M. Parental anticipatory mourning. In: Schoenberg B, Carr AC, Peretz D, Dutcher HH, eds. *Psychological Aspects of Terminal Care.* New York, NY: Columbia University

Press; 1972:42-52.

13. Meadows AT, Gordon J, Massari DS, Littman P, Ferguson J, Moss K. Declines in IQ scores and cognitive dysfunction in children with acute lymphocytic leukemia treated with cranial irradiation. *Lancet.* 1981;2:1015-1018.

14. Ross JW. The child with cancer in school. In: Fithian J, ed. *Understanding the Child with a Chronic Illness in the Classroom.* Phoenix, Ariz: Oryx Press;1984:152-272.

15. Ross JW, Disirens D, Turney ME. Evaluation of a symposium for educators of children with cancer. *J Psychosoc Oncol.* 1989;7:159-178.

16. Greer D et al., eds. *Final Report of the National Hospice Study.* Submitted to the Health Care Financing Administration, Washington, DC; 1984.

17. Rando TA. Bereaved parents: particular difficulties, unique factors and treatment issues. *Social Work.* 1985;30:19-23.

18. Cook JA, Wimberley DW. If I should die before I wake: religious commitment and adjustment to the death of a child. *J Scientific Study Religion.* 1983;915-922.

19. Ross JW. The role of the social worker with long-term survivors of childhood cancer and their families. *Social Work in Health Care.* 1982;7:1-13.

20. Zelter LK. The adolescent with cancer. In: Kellerman J, ed. *Psychological Aspects of Childhood Cancer.* Springfield, Ill: Charles C. Thomas; 1980:70-99.

21. Ross JW. Ethical conflicts in medical social work: pediatric cancer care as a prototype. *Health and Social Work.* 1982a;7:95-102.

22. Levy CS. *Social Work Ethics.* New York, NY: Human Science Press; 1976:79-93.

SOCIAL WORK SERVICES FOR THE CHILD AND FAMILY

Allison Stovall, MSW, CSW-ACP

INTRODUCTION

The diagnosis of cancer in childhood quickly involves the child, parents, and all family members in the complex world of present-day cancer treatment. In general, this world acknowledges the importance of treating the *child with a disease,* not just the disease itself. The child brings not only a biological reality to this world, but also a social and psychological one. The nature of the disease and the intensity of the treatment it requires produce physical, social, and emotional effects for the child, family, and society that demand attention.

In light of this awareness, medical and psychosocial team members share common and interrelated goals for patient and family: to preserve the life of the child and minimize suffering, while interfering as little as possible with normal growth and development; and to assist family system functioning so that the individual needs of family members can be met.

The enormity of these shared goals has led to the creation of multidisciplinary teams in most major medical centers. It is generally the clinical oncology social worker who is assigned major responsibility for assessing the psychosocial situation of the patient and family and for planning and delivering services to address the needs that are identified. In carrying out that responsibility, the social worker will assume many roles with patient and family: evaluator, counselor and/or therapist, educator, advocate, discharge planner, group worker, and liaison to hospital and community resources. In addition, professional concern for the needs of *all* the patients and families being served may lead to other roles: program planner, teacher, resource developer, researcher, and others.

Obviously, the ability to offer the array of social work services needed to assist children and families coping with childhood cancer depends not only on the clinical skills of the social worker, but also on knowledge about what pediatric patients and families generally must confront in dealing with a cancer diagnosis. With this knowledge, the social worker can then move to the critical tasks of assessing and planning interventions.

SCREENING ASSESSMENT OF PATIENTS AND FAMILIES

PURPOSE OF THE ASSESSMENT

The initial assessment process sets the stage for the development of a therapeutic relationship between the social worker and the family. It serves as the essential basis for the delivery of effective services and demonstrates to the child and family the importance the entire team of caregivers gives to understanding the impact of the cancer diagnosis on all family members. The social worker needs to gather pertinent facts about each family's life and convey that these facts will help team members work with child and family during the diagnostic work-up and throughout the treatment period.

It is often helpful to determine, at the outset, what the child and family understand about the reasons for a referral. Families arrive at the treatment center with different perceptions of the diagnostic information given by the referring physician. Social work assessment of these differing perceptions may help team members know what clarification is necessary.

While social workers can observe readily each family's way of managing during the crisis of the diagnostic phase, it is imperative to learn about the usual styles of coping and functioning of family members that existed prior to the diagnosis. Social workers need to know the strengths possessed by the child, the siblings, the parents, and other significant members of the family system. Observation of communication patterns provides information about the nature of family relationships. At the time of diagnosis, there may be a tendency for family members to protect each other because of the catastrophic fears often attached to the idea of cancer. Family members must be helped to understand the value of openness and honesty in addressing their questions.

The social worker must also obtain information on the family's socioeconomic status, which aids in evaluating family resources that can be tapped. Determination of educational and employment histories may help predict the possible reactions family members may encounter when the child's treatment disrupts school and work schedules. Such background information also helps staff anticipate family members' ability to understand relevant medical information. Exploration of economic resources available for covering the costs of treatment and the out-of-pocket expenses helps identify those families needing referral to financial assistance agencies. The family's prior experience with social agencies may help the clinician gauge how much assistance families may need in order to use such agencies in this new situation. It is helpful to learn about the degree of closeness within the family and friendship networks of a child who has become ill. These data help in predicting the tangible and emotional supports available to families struggling to achieve stability at a time of crisis. Exploration of formal and informal spiritual resources assists the social worker in understanding the family's values and beliefs as well as the meanings the family assigns to the occurrence of a serious, life-threatening, and chronic illness in their child. This knowledge also informs the social worker about perspectives family members bring to the process of making decisions affecting treatment. A complete assessment also takes into consideration the ethnic group to which the child and family belong. Membership in ethnic minorities may bring special viewpoints regarding illness that need to be understood by the health care team.

Each child and family facing the crisis of a cancer diagnosis require a psychosocial assessment if services are offered, but this therapeutic activity becomes essential for families who appear to be at high risk for having problems with basic social needs or in adaptation. During the screening process, which may begin with review of the patient's record, families who have financial needs, who have cognitive limitations, who must travel great distances to the treatment center, or whose primary language is not English should be noted. School and employment problems reported by the child and family generally will indicate a need for intervention. Unusual emotional responses on the part of the child or family members also warrant attention. Social workers must remember, however, that expressions of profound shock and anguish are common during the crisis phase of a cancer diagnosis, as parents begin to mourn the threatened loss of their child's life. Often, other members of the health care team may be alarmed at the initial behaviors of children and family members and may pressure the social worker to intervene in order to alter these behaviors quickly. Indeed, prolonged and severe emotional reactions of a child or family member usually require intervention. If examination of the family system reveals a lack of close family ties or a lack of open communication in the family, greater problems with adaptation are likely to emerge.

The gathering of this information is important because it provides the team of caregivers with an individualized picture of the child and family. The child is more than a victim of a dangerous disease. The child is a unique individual with special personal attributes who is developing socially within the context of a family, a school environment, and a home community. A thorough psychosocial assessment of the child and family can enhance the development of therapeutic relationships on the part of all team members. It can also aid in the development of an individualized and comprehensive treatment plan for the child that includes psychosocial interventions as well as medical ones.

HIGH-RISK SCREENING

Social workers with large caseloads may need to employ screening procedures to aid in setting priorities. These screening activities may lead to a social worker's emphasis on working with low-income families, single-parent or blended families, families belonging to ethnic minorities, or families with apparent difficulties in coping. Other high-risk families are those exhibiting extreme responses to diagnostic information and hospital routines, or those in which the patient is cognitively impaired.

FORMAT OF THE ASSESSMENT

The first section of the assessment should report the data gathered in the initial interviews, with careful delineation of what family members report about their personal situations.

This should include:

- Information on the structure of the nuclear and extended families and the composition of the household in which the child lives
- The sources of income and the employment histories of family wage earners
- The housing situation, noting the location of the home in relation to the treatment center and whether it is in an urban or rural setting

- Whether the dwelling is suitable for any specialized home care that may be needed in order to help the social worker anticipate discharge planning needs
- Descriptions of available support networks including neighbors, a community athletic team, the family's church, or the child's school
- Information on the child's level of academic performance and any changes that the child's parents or teachers may have noted just prior to diagnosis
- Assessment of the child's and family's attitudes toward informing the school of the child's medical situation.

These descriptive data should be followed by a section in which the social worker highlights the inherent strengths of the patient and family members and indicates how those strengths can help in developing positive ways of coping with the stresses imposed by the child's cancer. Problems or high-risk factors should be noted in this section. Finally, the assessment should include a list of the social worker's plans for the specific problems cited.

CLINICAL INTERVENTIONS WITH PATIENTS AND FAMILIES

CRISIS INTERVENTION

When parents learn that their child has cancer, they begin to experience loss of stability both individually and within the family system. This loss of internal and external balance constitutes the crisis situation characteristic of the diagnostic phase of the illness. Parents and other adults in the family become anxious about the possible loss of the child. The child's siblings worry about the sick brother or sister and resent the absence of their parents, even when they can understand the reasons for that absence. The anxieties of the patient vary with the child's age, but concerns about painful medical procedures, physical discomfort induced by treatment, and changes in appearance are common. The social worker can help the child and family recognize that the diagnosis of a severe, chronic illness can bring about upsetting feelings. Further intervention is directed at exploring and clarifying the feelings of each family member. Expression of fear, anger, and other common emotional responses can relieve the child and family members of some of their anxiety and feelings of hopelessness. In order to achieve the goal of crisis intervention–

restoring the family's level of functioning to that present prior to the crisis–the social worker must explore with the child and family their familiar coping styles. The social worker can help family members to understand how familiar coping mechanisms can be valuable in a new situation in which they may feel out of control, and to identify new ways of coping. When the patient's initial discharge from the hospital or clinic is imminent, the social worker can help the family members contemplate the activities and emotions connected with the return home. By rehearsing the possible reactions of family members, friends, and schoolmates, child and parents can feel more comfortable with the task of re-entry into the home community. The social worker needs to reinforce the fact that the child and family have learned important information about the illness.When the child returns for the first time to the treatment center, the crisis work can move to completion with a review of the ways in which the child and family members handled encounters with friends and relatives at home.

The process of crisis intervention is limited, but the social worker may employ it on a recurring basis when working with families. Even when the initial crisis of the diagnosis is substantially resolved, other crises may arise throughout the course of treatment. During maintenance therapy a crisis may ensue if a child requires surgery, especially if the situation arises from an emergency. A significant crisis can develop when the disease recurs, once a remission has been attained. When treatment has been successful and families face the termination of therapy, the patient and family may experience a crisis as they learn to function with much less dependency on the treatment center staff. At this juncture, the child and family must learn to cope with loss of the comfort they may have felt if they viewed therapy as minimizing the possibility of relapse. The most demanding crisis arises when staff must make the family aware that the child's cancer has progressed despite the use of proven therapeutic agents and that the child will die. These crisis periods can be helped to resolution by the same kinds of strategies employed during the crisis of diagnosis.

SUPPORTIVE COUNSELING

Throughout the course of treatment, the social worker may engage in an activity known as supportive counseling, which is aimed at maintaining the functional behaviors in all family members. Families may experience renewal of anxieties in anticipation of clinic visits, particularly in the early months of therapy. If the child receives some therapy from a physician close to home and therefore comes to the cancer center infrequently, then the return to the cancer center may induce even greater anxiety. Cancer is a chronic illness requiring some chronic adjustments as well. As part of ongoing work with child and family, the social worker needs to periodically review with them the tasks of adaptation. The social worker can help families anticipate problems that may arise as a result of changes within the family system or within the child and siblings as they undergo the processes of normal development. By maintaining an active interest in the successful adaptation of the child and family, the social worker demonstrates positive regard for them and their welfare. This enhances the individuals' feelings of worth and strengthens the therapeutic relationship. The social worker's efforts result in the family members feelings cared for and supported. When the social worker has taken the steps to establish a therapeutic relationship by offering such support, crisis work can be resumed more readily when necessary.

FAMILY COUNSELING

While the distance of the family's home from the treatment center often makes social work intervention with the family as a whole difficult, the social worker must keep the family context in mind when working with the child and available family members. Whether in a crisis phase of work with a family or when doing supportive counseling, the social worker must remember that all members of the family system feel the impact of the changes wrought when a child in the family has cancer. The social worker may bring family members together to address problems in communication, the need for expression of feelings, and confrontation of the effects of role realignments within the family. Such topics might be central themes in family therapy sessions in a mental health clinic as well. Typically, the family therapy practiced by a pediatric oncology social worker has the impact of the child's cancer as the underlying framework.

COLLABORATION WITH OTHER MENTAL HEALTH PROFESSIONALS

The degree to which social workers employ certain interventions depends, in part, on training and experience in specific areas. When staffing of the treatment center allows it, social workers may turn to other mental health professionals in the center to assist in working with the family. These include social workers who specialize in behavior therapy, individual psychotherapy, group work, or family therapy.

Many pediatric oncology social workers practice in university teaching hospitals and work with child-life specialists or recreation therapists in attending to the mental health needs of children and other family members. Social workers work well with these two disciplines and can act as mutual referral agents. The social worker in a pediatric oncology setting is child–and family–focused but may work most actively with the parents, especially if the patient is a preadolescent child. The child-life specialist may be aware of family issues but will use the media of play and activity to focus on work with the child.

Social workers assist physicians and nurses in identifying the need for neuropsychological assessment. The availability of psychologists in settings where children are treated for cancer varies greatly. Psychologists may be employed in pediatrics and, in many cases, are affiliated with the center's psychiatry department. This influences the working relationships between pediatric oncology social workers and clinical psychologists. In either situation, the social worker is the professional most likely to identify a need for psychological evaluation or intervention. The social worker may undertake the significant therapeutic task of preparing a child or family member for psychological counseling. If the psychologist is based in pediatrics, therapeutic work is more likely to be done conjointly by the social worker and a psychologist. In this situation, communication is likely to be enhanced.

CHILD MANAGEMENT INTERVENTIONS

The social worker's repertoire of interventions needs to include techniques aimed at modifying behaviors within the family. Parents possess a wide range of skills in managing their child's behavior. For some, positive nurturing skills that reinforce adaptive behavior come easily. Others employ practices that have negative repercussions. In working with the parents, social workers need to stress the importance of maintaining the normal limits used in family discipline prior to the diagnosis. Even parents who are aware of the importance of a consistent approach to family discipline may be tempted to overindulge a child with a serious illness. The social worker can assist parents in dealing with ambivalence about discipline by helping them to recognize that wanting to indulge the whims of a child with cancer is a normal response. Parents must be reminded, however, that singling out the child with cancer for special treatment is likely to disrupt normal development of each child in the family.

Parents may require assistance in talking with their children about cancer. Too often, fear about a possible fatal outcome will lead parents to protect their children, including the child with cancer, from medical information. Problems in this area surface when parents implore the health care staff to be less than forthright with the patient or the siblings regarding the diagnosis or prognosis. During maintenance therapy, these parents may be less than honest with their children regarding the scheduling of invasive procedures or of routine appointments. In these instances, the social worker needs to help parents confront the fears that underlie their reluctance to be honest with their children. The social worker can also assist the parents by advising them of several alternative ways of handling family communication related to the treatment process.

BEHAVIORAL TECHNIQUES

Social workers who are experienced in the behavioral techniques of desensitization, relaxation, and visual imagery can help a child who experiences anticipatory nausea and vomiting related to treatment, heightened anxiety over invasive medical procedures, or pain owing to surgery or progression of disease. Behavioral techniques serve to reduce anxiety, to distract from the perceived source of pain, to provide physical comfort, and to give the child greater feelings of control. Children as young as 7 years old may be good candidates for such interventions, provided that they have the skills necessary for benefitting from behavioral techniques.

EDUCATION

The educational activity of information sharing can enhance the sense of control needed by the child and family members. A preventive mental health model raises social workers' awareness that children and family members who are educated about cancer and treatment will feel more competent as they participate in treatment. The social worker can reinforce some of the educational messages of other team members including facts pertinent to the disease and the treatment process. It is important for social workers to educate families about the treatment center, as families will benefit from having information about the structure and function of a hospital. Families who receive information about resources both within the hospital and in the community tend to adapt more positively.

ADVOCACY

Social workers in pediatric oncology carry out advocacy activities, as they do in many other areas of the profession. Social workers serve as liaisons between family members and staff who may be having communication problems and who may hold conflicting views of the value of treatment. The social worker may assist parents in influencing treatment decisions involving their child by helping them prepare for conferences with the team and by helping to create opportunities for parents to be heard during such conferences.

Families may need the advocacy skills of a social worker when negotiating to secure needed services with representatives of various departments of the hospital and of community agencies. A child who is a patient in a comprehensive cancer center may encounter staff who are not fully sensitive to the needs of children in health care settings. They may be unnecessarily brusque with young patients or they may be insensitive to the child's need for parental presence in an area of the hospital where family participation is discouraged. The social worker can improve this situation by interpreting child and parental needs to personnel in areas outside of pediatrics where diagnostic or treatment procedures must be performed. Social workers also convey information about changes in family income or insurance status to the hospital business office or to community agencies, particularly those offering financial assistance. The special needs of chronically ill children may need to be advocated to public and private agencies when their guidelines for service seem inflexible.

GROUP WORK

Although social workers may concentrate on intervention with individuals or a particular family, some work with groups of children and families to assist them in adapting to the cancer experience. Groups may vary in structure, purpose, and focus. Groups based at the treatment center are more aptly called support groups rather than therapy groups. Their purpose is to help individuals strengthen their coping skills and to benefit from the experience of mutual support rather than to foster fundamental changes in personality structure. Various modes for structuring such groups are used. Children's groups may include patients and their siblings or separate groups for the two sets of children. Group interventions with children must vary according to ages and developmental levels of the members. Occasionally, a treatment center may have a large enough patient population to have a group for parents of new patients, but groups are usually composed of members with varying degrees of experience in dealing with cancer in their children. Some treatment centers offer groups for bereaved family members who may need a separate forum for addressing their special needs.

While groups that are billed as support groups may be threatening to some children, groups with an activity focus may have a wider appeal. Children may be able to lose themselves in a craft activity or a game and talk together about their experiences. Recreational activities designed for parents encourage mutual sharing. Programs aimed at fostering the enjoyment of family groups can reduce families' sense of social isolation.

Social workers may encounter family members, particularly parents, who embrace a self-help group model. While parents may want to set the agendas for such groups, they may want some assistance from the social worker based at the treatment center in locating speakers for program meetings. Social workers also serve as consultants to parents' groups regarding group formation and process. Affiliation with a hospital social worker may legitimize the self-help group in the eyes of the hospital staff.

SOCIAL WORKER ACTIVITIES THROUGHOUT TREATMENT PHASES

DISCHARGE PLANNING

Information obtained during the initial assessment that describes the household composition, the family and friendship support networks, and the distance of the home from the treatment center can assist the health care team in anticipating needs and making plans with the family at the time of discharge. The social workers' assessments of the family members' ability to comply with prescribed home care regimens also contributes to the discharge planning effort.

From the outset of a case, pediatric oncology social workers address the adaptations that family members and the new cancer patient must make when they return to the home community. Social workers help parents deal with anxieties about caring for their child at home where medical staff will not be as readily available as in the hospital. Families may also benefit from referrals to community support systems.

Case Management

In the role of case manager, social workers coordinate referrals to social support systems and to agencies that offer material assistance on the basis of needs assessments. While the child is treated in the hospital or in the outpatient clinic, the child and family establish ties with other families and form relationships with staff members. After discharge, affiliation with support groups in the community can reinforce the benefits of mutual sharing learned in the treatment center. The social worker can help family members identify the ways that such groups might be helpful, assist the family in locating the appropriate organizations, and follow up with the family on their use of these resources.

Early contacts should explore the kinds of financial assistance the family will need for meeting the costs of care. These costs include the expenses for medical treatment and the out-of-pocket costs of food, lodging, and transportation that accrue when the treatment center is some distance from the family's home. Referral to financial assistance agencies is a significant part of the social worker's contribution to discharge planning. In assuming the case manager's role, the social worker informs the family of the availability of financial assistance agencies, eligibility criteria, and the best ways to gain access to services. Parents are taught how to use these community resources and are followed up to determine whether the programs are meeting the family's needs. These referral activities aid families in feeling prepared for managing successfully at home following the child's discharge and they facilitate compliance with treatment regimens.

CONTINUITY OF CARE COORDINATION

In addition to ensuring that parents have the means to get their child to the treatment center, the social worker also may help facilitate the family's transfer to a medical facility nearer to their home. In this way the family gains comfort from knowing that the staff at the cancer center has good communication with the home-town team of caregivers who will take responsibility for monitoring the child's health, and often, for administering some of the therapy. The social worker can help the team in the home town respond to the family's needs by communicating to them the family's adaptation to the initial phase of treatment at the cancer center. When particular adjustment problems are cited, the hospital social worker may solicit the team's assistance in enlisting local mental health resources.

SCHOOL INTERVENTIONS

Some medical centers may include hospital teachers as part of the psychosocial team. They, along with the social workers and nurses, determine the child's current level of school activity with the intent of helping the child prepare to return to school following discharge from the cancer center. In some settings, this may be the task of the social worker. The social worker and family members can discuss options for preparing school personnel and classmates for the child's return to school. Parents may prefer to confer with the child's teacher and the school principal on their own or they may want the participation of personnel from the cancer center. Some children are comfortable helping teachers explain the illness to classmates, while others prefer that classmates be informed before they return. Social work intervention should focus on the development of open lines of communication among family members, school personnel, and the cancer center. Discussion of communication channels ensures greater likelihood that school personnel can create an individualized educational plan to accommodate the demands of ongoing treatment on the child.

In order to provide assistance with school re-entry issues, the social worker needs to collaborate with nurses, physicians, and teachers based at the cancer center. Pediatric oncology nurses can serve as effective liaisons with school nurses in working toward the goal of helping children resume normal school activity. School nurses unaccustomed to working with children with cancer can be educated by the pediatric oncology nurse regarding treatment and anticipated side effects. The nurses' interpretation of medical information can complement the social workers' communication with school personnel regarding adjustment issues. When the team includes hospital teachers, they can take the responsibility for discussing academic issues with personnel from the child's school. In some centers, a school coordinator is a team member who can take the lead in communication with the school using the social worker, the nurse, and the hospital teacher as resource people. Communication with the school takes place via telephone contacts, correspondence, and school visits. In some centers, team members have worked together to develop information packets and workshops for school personnel. When medical information is given to patients' schools or decisions are made about the timing of patients' re-entry into school, it is important that the pediatric oncologist participate as a consultant.

INTER-INSTITUTIONAL COLLABORATION

Another function of the social worker is to provide help to families who choose to consult other centers for second opinions or experimental therapy or who may be referred to other institutions for specialized treatment such as bone marrow transplant. When parents desire a second opinion regarding treatment for their child, the social worker can explore with the family their rationale for this and work with other team members to make necessary arrangements. In working with families who are searching for treatment alternatives, social workers must assure families that they support their right to seek this information. The social worker at the referring center can arrange for the family's contact with another social worker at the new institution, if this is desired.

When the family takes the child to another center for experimental therapy, the referring social worker can enhance the family's adaptation by establishing contact with the social worker whose team will be administering that therapy. This kind of social work intervention is significant when the patient will undergo bone marrow transplant or investigational treatment. The social worker at the receiving institution can be informative about transportation and housing resources as well as institutional procedures. The referring social worker can provide information on the family's coping skills that can assist the receiving social worker's efforts to aid them in their adjustment to the new center. A child and family who have great trust in the pediatric oncology team attending to them from the time of diagnosis may find it hard to transfer their trust to a new set of health care providers. The work of pediatric oncology social work colleagues on behalf of the family can enhance the parents' ability to make a successful transition at a critical stage in the child's treatment. This same kind of cooperative work between social workers is appropriate when a family needs to transfer a child's care to another hospital due to a geographic move. The family will receive comfort when the social worker at the referring institution makes follow-up contacts with them to check on the child's progress.

INTERVENTIONS BEYOND ACTIVE THERAPY

LONG-TERM SURVIVORS

After the completion of active therapy, children return to cancer centers for follow-up examinations and laboratory studies at lengthening intervals. Some institutions hold separate clinic sessions for the long-term survivors. In other settings, the child's primary pediatric oncologist continues this follow-up. Social workers' interventions with long-term survivors focus on supporting efforts to resume normal childhood activities. Social workers need to explore with children and their parents the progress made toward this goal, keeping in mind that some children may have trouble relinquishing the special status they may have attained in their families and their communities while they were on treatment. In addition to attending to developmental issues, social workers need to be aware of vocational and emotional rehabilitation to assist in dealing with the psychosocial sequelae of treatment. Former cancer patients still face discrimination from some employers and insurance providers and social workers need to be prepared to serve as patient advocates in these instances.

BEREAVED FAMILIES

A significant number of pediatric cancer patients die of the disease or of causes related to treatment. If families are willing to continue in counseling following a child's death, parents and siblings may be seen individually or in groups. For families who live a considerable distance from the cancer center, social workers can aid them in obtaining counseling locally. When counseling is not feasible because of logistics or reluctance to enter into scheduled counseling sessions, the social worker can set up a routine for follow-up telephone contacts. Parents need to know that the professionals who cared for their child have not forgotten them and are still interested in assisting them as they grieve the loss of their child. Some social workers supplement their contacts with families by supplying families with books or articles written to address bereavement issues.

PROGRAM AND POLICY DEVELOPMENT

As clinicians, social workers serve as direct advocates, a role also assumed when addressing the psychosocial needs of groups of patients and families. When it is clear to the social worker that families' needs are not being met, the social worker can work with other members of the team to design special programs. It may be necessary to interpret the needs of children to health care practitioners who do not have a pediatric focus by setting up a series of in-service programs. Often, this kind of interpretation is needed at facilities that are not devoted exclusively to the care of children.

As advocates for the consumers of health care services, social workers can design programs and develop or promote policies that include opportunities for patients and family members to offer their perspectives on health care delivery. Parents and patients may be invited to offer suggestions to committees that set policies for clinic and hospital operations or may serve as representatives to these committees. Some staff members may at times feel threatened by the presence of patients or parents in discussions of policy matters. Social workers may need to be assertive in speaking on behalf of consumers to these staff members.

Social workers can effectively serve families by assuming this kind of advocacy stance when participating in activities sponsored by voluntary health organizations or governmental agencies. Pediatric oncology social workers can offer knowledge of patients' and families' perspectives when working on the development of new programs with interested representatives of community agencies. Social workers also promote opportunities for the consumers of services to contribute directly to the formulation and implementation of policies that affect their welfare.

When pediatric oncology social workers learn of programs in other locales that might be of benefit to clients of their centers, they can facilitate the adaptation of the programs to the needs of these families. Social workers may serve as consultants to self-help groups such as affiliates of the Candlelighters Childhood Cancer Foundation or they may devise programs designed to enhance families' adaptation to childhood cancer after learning of innovative programs designed by social work colleagues. Social workers may choose to concentrate on adaptation issues of special interest to them in program development activities.

COMMUNITY EDUCATION

Social workers engage in a variety of community educational efforts either individually as representatives of the institutions where they are employed or as committee members with voluntary health agencies.

Social workers may preside at educational sessions where families are given information about positive ways of coping with the cancer experience. They may collaborate with other health care providers to develop patient education materials within individual institutions or as part of broader educational efforts sponsored by voluntary health care organizations.

Pediatric oncology social workers also participate in activities directed to the public and the professional community as members of professional organizations such as ACCH (Association for the Care of Children's Health), APOSW (Association of Pediatric Oncology Social Workers), and NAOSW (National Association of Oncology Social Workers). They contribute to professional educational efforts by writing for journals and developing professional educational materials.

TEACHING RESPONSIBILITIES

By combining theoretical knowledge, clinical experience, and research findings regarding families' experience with childhood cancer, pediatric oncology social workers serve informally and formally as educators for fellow professionals and members of other disciplines. Social workers provide orientation sessions for members of other disciplines when they join the team in a pediatric cancer treatment center. These sessions cover the dynamics of the childhood cancer experience and explain the social work role in helping children and families cope with cancer. Similar sessions may be held for residents, medical students, and other trainees who rotate through teaching hospitals. Primarily, social workers provide clinical teaching while engaged in the delivery of social work services. In some instances, social workers may have opportunities to participate in more formal educational forums such as courses presented in schools that train health care professionals. By serving as field instructors for graduate social work students, clinical social workers help increase the ranks of professionals with the specialized knowledge needed for working with children who have cancer.

SUMMARY

In their work with children with cancer, social workers come to know families in crisis. Social workers draw from the knowledge base that is the foundation of the profession to help these families cope with the impact of having seriously ill children, and from knowledge about childhood cancer and its treatment. Social workers direct their efforts at helping families successfully integrate the experience of childhood cancer into their lives with minimal disruption. Cancer strikes at peoples' most profound emotions and treasured values, thereby making it difficult for families to achieve the goal of successfully coping with the cancer experience. Pediatric oncology social workers can enhance work toward that goal by offering their knowledge of family functioning, their experience with appropriate helping techniques, and their compassion.

SUGGESTED READINGS

Adams DW, Deveau EJ. *Coping with Childhood Cancer.* Reston,Va: Reston Publishing Co; 1984.

Adams-Greenley M. Psychological staging of pediatric cancer patients and their families. *Cancer.* 1986;58:449-453.

Adams-Greenley M, Shiminaki-Maher T, McGowan N, Meyers PA. A program for helping siblings of children with cancer. *J Psychosoc Oncol.* 1986;4:55-67.

Bloom BS, Knorr RS, Evans AE. The epidemiology of disease expenses. *JAMA.* 1985;253:2393.

Cairns NU, Clark GM, Smith SD, Lansky SB. Adaption of siblings to childhood malignancy. *J Pediatr.* 1979; 95:484-487.

Carr-Gregg M, White L. Siblings of pediatric cancer patients: a population at risk. *Med Pediatr Oncol.* 1987;15:62-68.

Chesler MA, Barbarin OA. *Childhood Cancer and the Family.* New York, NY: Brunner/Mazel; 1987.

Christ G, Adams MA. Therapeutic strategies at psychosocial crisis points in the treatment of childhood cancer. In: *Childhood Cancer–Impact on the Family.* New York, NY: Plenum Press; 1984.

Copeland DR, Pfefferbaum B, Stovall AJ. *The Mind of the Child Who Is Said to be Sick.* Springfield, Ill: Charles C. Thomas; 1983.

Futterman EH, Hoffman I. Crisis and adaptation in the families of fatally ill children. *The Child in His Family: The Impact of Disease and Death.* New York, NY: John Wiley & Sons; 1973.

Gogan JL, Koccher GP, Foster DJ, O'Malley JE. Impact of childhood cancer on siblings. *Health and Social Work.* 1977; 2:41-57.

Kagen-Goodheart L. Re-entry: living with childhood cancer. *Am J Orthopsychiatry.* 1977; 47:4.

Kellerman J. Comprehensive psychological care of the child with cancer: description of a program. In: *Psychological Aspects of Childhood Cancer.* Springfield, Ill: Charles C. Thomas; 1980.
Kellerman J, ed. *Psychological Aspects of Childhood Cancer.* Springfield, Ill: Charles C. Thomas; 1980.
Koch-Hattem A. Siblings' experience of pediatric cancer: interviews with children. *Health and Social Work.* 1986;107-117.
Lansky SH. Management of stressful periods in childhood cancer. *Pediatric Clin North Am.* 1985;32:625-632.
Lauria MM. Family adaption to childhood cancer: a clinical perspective. In: *Proceedings of the National Conference on Practice, Education and Research in Oncology Social Work–1984.* New York, NY: American Cancer Society; 1985.
Ross JW. Social work intervention with families of children with cancer. *Social Work in Health Care.* 1978; 7:1-13.
Ross JW, Scarvalone SA. Facilitating the pediatric cancer patient's return to school. *Social Work.* 1982; 27:256-61.
Schulman JL, Kpst MJ. *The Child with Cancer.* 1980.
Sourkes BM. Siblings of the pediatric cancer patient. *Psychological Aspects of Childhood Cancer.* Springfield, Ill: Charles C. Thomas; 1980.
Spinetta JJ, Deasy-Spinetta P, eds. *Living with Childhood Cancer.* St. Louis, Mo: CV Mosby; 1981.

SPECIAL PROGRAMS FOR CHILDREN WITH CANCER AND THEIR FAMILIES

Nancy F. Cincotta, MSW, CSW, ACSW, CCLS

SPECIAL PROGRAMS

Childhood cancer is emotionally, physically, and financially demanding on the entire family, but often, the negative impact of the illness can be minimized through special programs in pediatric oncology. These programs, which primarily come under the auspices of hospitals and the community of cancer organizations, offer unique services to patients and their families. At critical stages during a child's treatment, a trip to camp or arrangements for a family member to stay at a Ronald McDonald House can alleviate stress and lessen the burden of the disease.

The social worker has varied roles in these special programs. In certain settings, the social worker's charge is to establish a special program to meet an identified need, but more often it is the social worker's role to accurately assess a family's specific needs at a given point in treatment and to make a referral to an appropriate program. Networking with other social workers through groups such as the Association of Pediatric Oncology Social Workers (APOSW) or the National Association of Oncology Social Workers (NAOSW) is vital to learning about existing resources. Additionally, contact with community organizations that serve cancer patients is invaluable. Whether a program is designed to provide respite, education, socialization, therapy, fun, or some combination of these, its positive impact should not be minimized. Often, such special programs are highlights of children's and parents' experiences during cancer treatment.

Because childhood cancers affect the entire family, special programs are created to meet the needs of patients and to address the concerns of siblings, parents, or the family as a whole. Whether establishing needs or making referrals to special programs, the social worker must consider the stage of illness, the child's strengths and limitations, and the family's financial and emotional status. Special programs offer families and patients opportunities to share information, thoughts, and experiences that will enable them to cope with feelings of depression, isolation, and immobilization.

CAMP PROGRAMS

Summer camp affords children a nurturing, recreational environment in which to develop skills and relationships. Children with cancer have fewer opportunities to experience such routine activities of childhood. In recognition of the need for both socialization and normalization, a variety of camp programs for children with cancer have been established. These programs are positive experiences that allow children to engage in age-appropriate activities and to interact with other children who are ill and have had experiences in common. These attributes of camp can help foster self-esteem and normal development. The side effects of rigorous treatment protocols may limit a child's regular opportunities for socialization with peers or time away from parents. Friendships made at cancer camps become important to children and can be helpful to them long after the camping season is over.

Camps exclusively for children with cancer provide environments in which to engage in physical activities, for some the first time since diagnosis. Children who have become cancer patients have the opportunity to master skills (e.g., boating, swimming) of which they have not previously felt capable. Children, as well as their parents, may approach the idea of camp with a mixture of enthusiasm and understandable apprehension. Through discussion of concerns, the social worker can help initially reluctant parents and prospective campers recognize that camp can be a safe setting, especially since there are on-site medical services and other support services. Some camps offer separate weekend programs for parents to attend during their child's stay. With support and encouragement, camp can be a therapeutic experience for all.

While some camp programs offer sessions exclusively for children with cancer, others provide experiences for children and their siblings, and still others involve the entire family. The choice can depend on individual family needs at a given time and the availability of specific programs. For example, a young adolescent, struggling with an increasingly dependent role because of the illness, may benefit from the independence of a camp setting.

Camp programs give parents a respite from their daily routines and help them to understand that their child can function independently (in the company of responsible adults). These programs also serve to provide parents time to attend to their own needs and desires. A camp experience serves as a reminder of a world that exists beyond cancer. It can be the perfect escape from the intensity of treatment. This time away from the medical setting can help families refocus and replenish their energies, or it can simply be a well-deserved vacation for everyone.

Camp programs are sponsored by a variety of organizations, usually without cost to the family. However, the cost of transportation to and from camp may impede the ability of some to participate. Hospital social work departments or community agencies may have special funds to assist with meeting these costs. Camp is an enriching experience that should be accessible to all eligible children and their families.

RONALD MCDONALD HOUSES

Ronald McDonald Houses started with one house in Philadelphia and now exist nationally. These Houses are perhaps the best known of the special programs for children with cancer. Pediatric cancer patients and their families can stay at these Houses during the course of inpatient and outpatient treatment. This is particularly helpful if the family's home is a considerable distance from the treatment center or if the child is critically ill. At times when the child is hospitalized and only one person can stay in the hospital, the other parent (and a sibling) may stay at a Ronald McDonald House. In certain situations such as bone marrow transplantation, during which a parent may not be permitted to remain in the hospital, the family's stay at Ronald McDonald House can facilitate daily visiting. When the child who has undergone transplantation is an outpatient, a Ronald McDonald House stay often makes it easier to return to the hospital quickly if a crisis occurs.

Some Ronald McDonald Houses have affiliated professional psychosocial staff to provide support services. The oncology social worker often serves as liaison to the House, referring families, assessing the family's ability to pay a minimal amount for their lodging, and making recommendations to the House managers. For those from other countries, it may be at the Ronald McDonald House that family members begin to learn crucial information about this country.

The Houses operate on a communal living model in which living, dining, kitchen, and sometimes, bathroom space is shared. Parents cook for themselves and are assigned cleaning tasks. At times, House staff members orchestrate special events such as parties and holiday activities.

SCHOOL PROGRAMS

School is the workplace of the child. Once a child reaches a certain age, societal expectations are that the child will be enrolled in an academic program. School provides an environment for learning and for socializing. If school attendance loses importance after diagnosis, the child may conclude that he or she is gravely ill. Missing school denies a child age-appropriate opportunities for continued intellectual and emotional growth and development. Whether a child likes school or not, or whether or not the child performs well in school, most children recognize that school is something in which they must participate and something that everyone their age does. Integrating school in the child's life at a time when a family is in the middle of a crisis challenges everyone involved.

The family's and the child's feelings about school prior to diagnosis will play a role in their responses to school after diagnosis. A child who never liked school before is unlikely to be excited about returning to school and may see the illness as an opportunity to avoid it. A child who enjoyed school and misses the experience may have an easier period of reacclimation.

Returning to school after the period of diagnosis and initial treatment can be traumatic for a child. Feelings of anxiety over seeing peers or teachers again and feelings of confusion about who and what to tell about their illness are common. Parents as well as children will need help as they prepare for a child's return to school. An innovative videotape, "Why, Charlie Brown? Why?" is available through the American Cancer Society. It is useful in helping families deal with these issues. Many medical centers and local organizations also have helpful videotapes about school re-entry which they sell, lend, or rent.

Most children fear that they will be ridiculed because of their appearance and feel anxious about what they have missed. If they are not feeling well, they may worry about keeping up with the demands of their school work. The need for periodic absences may be stressful and may also impede learning. When indicated and available, adjunctive tutoring can be helpful.

In addition to the recognized value of the school experience for a child on treatment, teachers, peers, and a structured day can provide support, encouragement, and diversion. Whenever possible, returning to school is usually the best alternative for the young patient.

Certain types of cancer require rigorous protocols that may involve prolonged hospitalization, during which time children may be so ill that they are unable to attend school. In these cases, local boards of education will provide tutoring after receiving documentation from the treatment center specifying the child's specific limitations. Many treatment centers have on-site academic programs for pediatric patients. Some have a schoolroom within the medical unit. Another option is individual tutoring on a daily basis or as the child's condition warrants.

For children who are unable to return to school, ongoing contact with school staff and classmates will help them remain connected to their classes and friends. Visits, cards, and homework assignments will enable the child to remain optimistic about returning to school at a later time. A child who is kept informed about school activities will feel less anxiety over what is being missed. Encouraging visits from a school counselor or teacher who knows the child can also be helpful.

Understanding and dealing with cancer or other severe illness in the classroom can be a difficult issue. Many pediatric oncology centers offer training sessions for school staff to learn about the physical and emotional aspects of childhood cancer. Health care personnel are in a unique position to offer vital information. This type of program can help school staff maximize their ability to help pediatric cancer patients. In this milieu informed professionals can also explore and deal with any anxiety that the school staff have about an ill child's return to school. Some treatment centers have school visiting programs in which members of the child's treatment team go to the school and meet with the teacher, the nurse, the class, or an assembly of children, depending on the needs and wishes of the school and family.

GROUP WORK SERVICES

Historically, group work has been an avenue used by social workers for offering assistance to persons faced with similar, difficult situations.

Groups can offer children with cancer and their family members the opportunity to share their own illness-related experiences and learn from the experiences of others. The social worker, alone or with other team members, can play various roles in relation to groups offered in a particular institution or community. The social worker can:

- Assess the need for a particular hospital-based group, design it, and provide leadership for it (e.g., monthly sibling group)
- Help facilitate the development of a self-help group (e.g., a Candlelighters group)
- Design and serve as facilitator for a group that addresses a specific need (i.e., coming off treatment, limited session group)
- Serve as planner, leader, or facilitator for community-based groups, that often are under the auspices of local units of the American Cancer Society or chapters of the Leukemia Society of America.

Groups can target patients, parents, siblings, or families; be planned for particular age groups (e.g., play or activity groups for preschoolers or younger children to help them deal with surgery or painful procedures, or adolescent groups to encourage peer discussion of treatment experiences); or be designed to address the changing issues of different treatment phases (e.g., groups for parents of newly diagnosed children, for learning stress management, for dealing with bereavement or post-treatment concerns). Groups can be time-limited (for a fixed number of sessions), open-ended, or one-time events. They can also take the form of generalized support and/or educational groups without any predetermined agenda. They may meet in inpatient, outpatient, or community settings during the day or in the evenings. The time (e.g., evening, weekend, afternoon), a group is offered will automatically make it accessible to some while excluding others (e.g., working parents).

While groups can supplement more individually tailored interventions with children and families, participation should be by invitation rather than expectation. Interest in group involvement on the part of child, parent, or sibling is not always universal. The value that groups offer to many must not obscure the fact that individual needs and preferences should be respected. At certain stages families may be more open to group work services than others. For children and family members who are amenable to group work services, such programs can afford them immeasurable support and strength.

CANDLELIGHTERS

Candlelighters is a national foundation established in 1970 by parents of cancer patients to advocate for the needs of children with cancer and to foster communication among parents. Many parent support groups have been established under its auspices nationwide and in foreign countries. The national office can refer a parent to groups or contact people in a specific area. The aim of parents helping parents is to empower the parent through mutual support and to disseminate information and resources. Parents who travel far from home to get to the treatment center, who are interested in peer support, or who are uncomfortable participating in a hospital-based group, might benefit from participation in a self-help community Candlelighters group.

In some areas, a hospital social worker serves as co-leader or consultant to the Candlelighters group. Each Candlelighters group is different, as membership and activities vary from community to community.

Candlelighters, with financial assistance from the American Cancer Society, publishes two quarterly magazines, one for teenagers and one for parents and professionals. These contain information of interest to patients, parents, siblings, and all who have contact with children with cancer. Patients who are reluctant to talk about their treatment may benefit from reading about someone else's feelings or experiences. These newsletters provide parents and children with helpful ideas on how to communicate with one another. Children can find a pen pal through the newsletter. This may be particularly significant for a child who is inactive or temporarily bedridden due to the illness.

SOCIAL WORK ORGANIZATIONS

The Association of Pediatric Oncology Social Workers (APOSW) is a membership organization of pediatric oncology social workers throughout the United States and Canada, with some members from other countries. The members of this organization can provide a wealth of information and support to the new worker in pediatric oncology. An annual conference and a quarterly newsletter are offered.

The National Association of Oncology Social Workers (NAOSW) is an organization of social workers from the United States and Canada, with some members from other countries. This organization provides the same services as the APOSW, but includes social workers who work with adults as well.

Membership and committee involvement in professional organizations can provide the social worker with support and opportunities to maximize skills in a demanding field through networking and education. Resources that help professionals maintain themselves in oncology social work are crucial. Although some social workers are in hospitals or organizations that have a built-in structure for support and education, there is additional benefit that can be gained from peer involvement with these national organizations.

DREAM/WISH PROGRAMS

The granting of a wish, something a child would like to have or do, can be a very special event in the child's life, especially in the context of illness. Numerous organizations throughout the United States grant wishes. The criteria for eligibility vary greatly. Some offer their services only to children who are "terminally ill," while others serve children at any stage of chronic illness. The criterion of terminal illness does not mean that death must be imminent, but rather that relapse or recurrence signals that the prognosis has worsened.

Some wish programs operate nationally with local chapters. Others are community-based. Before a social worker refers a family to a wish organization, it is important to determine whether the child fits that group's criteria. Even the quietest child can become excited at the prospect of choosing and planning a wished-for experience or item, and unnecessary disappointment for the child, family, and staff should be avoided.

Generally, these organizations stipulate that a child cannot receive a wish from more than one program. Some treatment centers have their own funds to provide an item or trip that a child desires, but these programs are not considered "formal" wish organizations and may not make a child ineligible for another program. Often, financial restrictions are placed on the total cost of the wish. This limit and similiar restrictions on the number of people who can be involved in the child's wish vary from organization to organization. Such stipulations need to be discussed with and understood by the family from the outset.

The experience of receiving a present or trip during a time that may be perceived as one in which options and control are limited by illness can boost morale. The value of giving a child with cancer the freedom to choose something special, ranging from a video casette recorder to a grand piano, or a trip to Disney World, cannot be underestimated. The social worker should be aware of strategic times during the course of treatment to consider referral to a wish program. The wish can be an adjunct to treatment, revitalizing the family and helping them to endure negative aspects of the illness.

When a child is terminally ill, however, the considerations are different. The family, and perhaps the child, may see the wish as a last request. Careful consideration of the child's limitations and capabilities are crucial. Under these circumstances, the wish will provide the family with something to plan and look forward to at a time when they feel hopeless. Frequently, the wish will be among the last happy memories a family can create together and therefore becomes precious. In addition to the benefit from the actual experience, the child and family also have the opportunity to enjoy the excitement of planning and then the joy of reliving the experience.

Some organizations do not provide individual gifts during the year but may solicit children's wishes for "things" and then provide them at a holiday party in December. Staff at the American Cancer Society, at Ronald McDonald Houses, or other social workers in the community can inform new social workers of such programs. A referral to a wish organization can be a very rewarding experience for a new social worker. In this task, the social worker becomes the conduit to the wish, the person who enables the family to have a positive experience that is not focused on the illness. (See Resource chapter for more information on specific programs).

FUN/SOCIALIZATION PROGRAMS

Cancer treatment is very demanding and stressful. Programs focused on fun can help patients, families, and staff have an event to plan and anticipate. These events include picnics, holiday parties, outings to sports events, masquerade parties, and others.

Children have special events in their lives that are not related to their illness. It is important to work with families to help children maintain a role in the activities that are important to them such as birthday parties, proms, and graduations.

HOSPICE PROGRAMS

The impending death of a child is always a difficult period. The choice of whether a child will die at home, in the hospital, or in an inpatient hospice unit is a very personal one. This is a decision made by the family and members of the health care team. The decision may be influenced by the availability of services in a particular community.

A family's choice may depend on the amount of support that is available at home, the ages and the needs of other children, religious perspective, or the child's wishes. Feelings about this choice may fluctuate and options should remain available even after a decision is made. If there is a prolonged period from the time death seems imminent and when it occurs, additional social work or in-home nursing services may be required.

BEREAVEMENT PROGRAMS

As family members and professional staff struggle to cope with the death of a child, bereavement programs offer individuals the opportunity to share and legitimize their thoughts and feelings. Bereavement services can be offered on an individual, group, or family basis and may be hospital- or community-based. For some parents, returning to the treatment center is too painful and they will not attend a group that meets on hospital grounds. Others find comfort in returning to the familiar environment of the hospital. Still others view returning to the hospital as something they must master in order to move on.

Bereavement groups can be time-limited, or ongoing with closed or open membership. The structure will depend on the auspices under which the program is offered or on the particular goal of the group. A time-limited model generally focuses on helping a number of parents at a similar stage get through the initial tasks of bereavement. Ongoing groups with open membership may function as an environment in which parents can help one another over time to recognize and deal with the various stages and tasks associated with surviving the loss of a child. Social workers involved in bereavement groups should be aware that some groups will need help in ending, once group members have moved toward resolution of psychosocial issues. Compassionate Friends, a national organization with local chapters, is a self help group for parents who have lost children to illness, accident, or suicide. These groups do not have leaders, so the tenor of the group varies according to who comprises its membership at a given time. This can be a useful resource if parents want exclusively a peer support group or in locations where no other support groups exist.

In order to administer a bereavement group, there must be a large number of bereaved parents who potentially would participate. Unless the social worker is employed in an organization that services a significant number of bereaved persons, it is often fruitful to have these services provided in the community or cooperatively among several organizations. Bereavement programs that are not hospital-based may be run by cancer organizations, social service agencies, hospices, counseling centers, or religious groups. It is important to remember that parents are not alone in their grief. Siblings and other family members should be considered for referral to appropriate services.

MEMORIAL SERVICES

Memorial services, often held at the hospital, can serve as a means to assist in the grieving process. After a child dies, the family, friends, and professional staff may feel the need for some type of conclusion to a patient's life, beyond the funeral service. A family may wish to have a memorial event, some time after the funeral, to share memories and feelings with others in a way they were unable to do soon after the death.

Medical staff members may express desires to acknowledge the lives and deaths of particular children. In these cases, they may or may not choose to invite families, depending on whether they wish to have a private remembrance. A service at the hospital chapel or a conference or team meeting concerning the child can serve this need. Some institutions hold monthly chapel services to acknowledge the children who died during the preceding month.

Several centers have periodic memorial or remembrance programs. Parents and other family members are invited back annually (or biannually) for an event such as a program of speakers or a luncheon. The purposes of these programs are to acknowledge the continued caring for these families, to recognize the communal sense of loss for staff and families, and to offer an opportunity for families to network. These programs can be difficult to plan, owing to the intensity of feelings evoked by bringing together a large number of families of children who have died.

CONCLUSION

The pediatric oncology social worker must consider many aspects of program development for children with cancer and their family members. Limited resources of personal and institutional time, money, staff, patient population, or interest may impede the ability to develop particular programs. Frequently, referral to an outside program is precisely what is indicated or is the only feasible plan. Collaborative efforts between the hospital and community agencies enable maximum service provision to this unique patient population.

Many organizations such as the Leukemia Society of America and the American Cancer Society offer educational materials and counselling services and also advocate for pediatric patients at local and national levels. Sharing the commitment in offering service to this special group of children and their families often affords the clinician a greater capability to meet their many needs. A strategic referral to an appropriate special program can be therapeutic for the family and professionally gratifying to the social worker. Childhood cancer is a demanding illness, creating multiple needs that can best be met through diverse programs.

PROFESSIONAL ISSUES IN ONCOLOGY SOCIAL WORK

Naomi M. Stearns, MSW, LICSW

INTRODUCTION

Working with cancer patients and their families can be one of the most professionally stimulating and rewarding experiences of a social worker's career. As patients and families confront the daily challenges posed by a chronic, life-threatening illness, they are generally receptive to social work involvement. The majority of social workers providing services to cancer patients do not practice in cancer centers or in major teaching hospitals; in fact, most do not work exclusively with cancer patients. However, it is safe to suggest that all social workers, regardless of the setting in which they practice, will at some time during their careers have the opportunity and challenge of dealing with cancer patients and/or their families. For this reason it is useful for social workers to become familiar with the emergent professional issues that have an impact on practice.

In recent years, treatment options have expanded and the survival rates for many cancer patients have increased. In addition, economic factors that influence funding, staffing, and reimbursement have changed the way health care is delivered. Each of these changes continues to have a major impact on oncology social work practice. The social work role has expanded to meet the increased demands imposed by more complex treatment modalities and shrinking resources.

A number of professional issues have surfaced as oncology social work has evolved as a specialty. Some might seem, at first glance, to relate only to social workers practicing in large medical settings or cancer research centers. However, all social workers who see cancer patients, regardless of the setting, need to be knowledgeable about these rapid changes and the concerns they raise for patients, families, and their caregivers.

In addition to the core knowledge about the impact of medical illness, oncology has its own vocabulary and unique qualities. There are many ways to develop clinical expertise in oncology, experience being the best teacher. Social workers can read numerous professional texts, as well as a plethora of first-person accounts of the cancer experience. Several cancer centers offer clinical skills courses in oncology social work that range in length from several days to a week. Additional information about skill building will be addressed later in this chapter.

COLLABORATION

The team delivery of health care is never more crucial than in oncology, and the concept raises numerous professional issues regarding collaboration. Twenty years ago, cancer researchers who treated patients may or may not have included a social worker on their relatively small team. Today, few would question the wisdom and appropriateness of having a social worker on the team. The ACCC (Association of Community Cancer Centers) originally articulated a standard for social work services, stating that "qualified individuals provide social work services to meet the psychosocial needs of patient/families." More recently, the National Association of Oncology Social Workers (NAOSW) developed its own standards of practice (see Appendix I) that are applicable to social work practice within cancer centers and teaching and community hospitals. Even in hospitals where social work departments are being reduced, cancer patients and their families are expected to receive social work services. This places the social worker in a unique position on the team, but it also raises questions regarding role differentiation and expectations about who should provide what to patients and families. The social worker frequently is the pivotal person in facilitating continuity of care in a system where so many professionals provide that care. Social workers who are cognizant of the potential for fragmentation are in a unique position to use their skills to increase communication among team members.

Educating others on the team about the diversity of the social work role can be challenging and at times frustrating. The perceptions of others on the health care team generally define their expectations of social work and influence their understanding of what it offers patients and families. Social workers whose major function is discharge planning may feel that their clinical assessment and therapeutic skills are not fully appreciated; social workers who are considered part of the mental health team are often perceived as lacking adequate understanding of the patient's practical needs. While social workers might feel the need to explain to others what professional education and skills they possess, the most effective way to demonstrate those abilities is by example. By demonstrating knowledge of and respect for the integration of the biological, psychological, social, and practical needs of cancer patients and their families, the social worker is able to provide a model for patient care. Tensions within the team are bound to surface, especially in times of shrinking resources and growing demands on staff energies.

Turf issues present yet another arena for professional conflict. In any multidisciplinary setting there are bound to be some conflicts. While a certain amount of team tension can be stimulating and healthy, it is important to separate the administrative issues from those related to the emotional intensity of the work itself. A work environment that respects the emotional drain on its staff and that encourages professional development among its team members certainly enhances everyone's ability to continue to function effectively.

ETHICAL ISSUES

Oncology social workers have major concerns regarding the ethics of cancer care. They are involved on a daily basis with issues of truth telling, patient autonomy, self-determination, informed consent, and quality of life. Cancer diagnosis and treatment have spawned ongoing debates around disclosure, randomized clinical trials, curative vs. palliative care (treatment oriented to symptom management), appropriate limits of treatment, and orders not to resuscitate. New workers, in particular, are forced to define and confront on a daily basis the concept of a "burdensome" life. In oncology practice, professional staff often find themselves grappling with competing values. Certain patient care decisions may threaten to force the caregivers to compromise their integrity. Social workers are particularly vulnerable in situations where treatment choices appear to undermine patient autonomy. Self-determination has been the foundation of social work training; as technology advances, the burden of choice increases. Patients are forced to consider the tradeoff between high-tech medical treatments, such as bone marrow transplantation and biological therapies, and what they and their families consider an acceptable quality of life or death.

The social worker frequently is asked to assist patients in sorting out the treatment options presented to them by the physician. One soon learns just how difficult the choices can be. Adjuvant treatment for breast cancer is but one example of this type of dilemma for patients for whom the options may seem confusing. In general, there is much controversy within the medical community regarding the "best treatment" for breast cancer. How does the patient choose? A dilemma arises for social workers when they feel pressure to support a specific treatment, especially when its benefit for the patient is unclear. One current debate centers on the use of biotherapeutics, in which patients essentially pay for their own research. This is a controversial issue with no easy answers. Maintaining a neutral stance can be difficult and, at times, inappropriate.

Communication between the physician and social worker is essential. The social worker's role in the patient-physician relationship must be clarified and the physician should keep the social worker apprised of what information the patient has been given. Having a social worker present during physician-patient discussions allows all participants to hear what the physician tells the patient about proposed treatments and possible side effects, both medical and psychosocial. It also helps social workers identify areas that need further explanation by the physician in order to facilitate the patient's decision-making process. The social worker's presence also allows observation of the interaction between the patient and physician and the patient and family, which helps in understanding how information is being given and received. Including social workers in such meetings enhances their credibility as vital members of the team.

Other ethical conflicts relate to the social worker's expectations regarding the goal of treatment. While one might prefer to think in terms of cure, it is helpful to understand that, at times, cure is not the objective, despite the aggressiveness and difficulty of the treatment. Frequently, treatment is an attempt to both manage the symptoms and maximize the quality of the patient's life within the constraints imposed by the disease, or perhaps, to think in terms of slowing down a terminal process when that is consistent with the patient's goals. An untreated cancer can cause serious disruptions of bodily functions and for that reason alone, palliative treatment is often recommended.

The issue of self-determination, a basic principle in the generic practice of social work, is highlighted in every discussion of ordinary vs. extraordinary means. Do-not-resuscitate orders, living wills, and artificial feeding are among the most commonly debated issues of self-determination in cancer care. Self-determination is a professional issue that social workers are well-equipped to debate, but one that often creates anxiety for the staff as they try to interpret patients' and families' wishes and concerns to the other members of the team. This is especially true when the patient's desires conflict with those of the family or those of the physician.

New legislation should encourage earlier discussions about patients' wishes and provide direction to family members and staff. The Patient Self Determination Act became effective nationwide in December 1991. The Act mandates that all hospitals, HMOs, and nursing homes that receive Medicare and Medicaid reimbursements provide written information to patients regarding their rights to refuse care, to create Advance Care Directives, and to appoint agents (proxies) to make decisions for them should they become unable to do so. It is important to know the way this policy is being carried out in one's work setting, where applicable, and how the social workers are involved.

When considering these ethical issues, a frequent concern is whether medicine has the right to create a "burdensome" life with its interventions. How does one define "burdensome?" What may seem to the medical team to be rather ordinary medical intervention may seem to certain patients radical or extraordinary and, indeed, burdensome in their own circumstances. The terminology used in discussing professional ethical issues is often vague. The term "heroic measures," for example, is wide open to interpretation. It is necessary to find out the patient's interpretation of the word. The physician's interpretation is equally important. While one physician might consider admission to an intensive care unit an heroic step, another might interpret cardiopulmonary resuscitation as routine, rather than heroic. Discussions about prognosis can be extremely misleading, as even the most considered medical prognostication is cloaked in uncertainty. Social workers and others on the health care team must understand the impracticality of absolute prognoses.

In most medical settings there is a tendency to generalize and often decisions reflect what is more convenient or less disruptive for the hospital than for the patient and family. Ethical practice dictates that care be individualized. While this is sound conceptually, it may be difficult institutionally. One of social work's goals is to return to patients some of the control they relinquish upon entering a medical setting. This particular issue should be of utmost concern to oncology social workers.

It is important for social workers to be in basic agreement with the philosophy of the institution in which they work. For example, social workers in cancer research centers soon learn that they work in an environment where there is generally always another treatment to be tried when one treatment fails to elicit a favorable response. That kind of aggressive approach may provoke quality-of-life issues for social workers new to the field. It is important that social workers allow enough time to fully understand an institution's orientation so that they can make informed judgments about their ability to fit in. Each of us brings to our work a set of beliefs and values that influence our handling of ethical dilemmas. It is important to understand that all medical decisions ultimately are made by two or more persons, each with his or her own moral and ethical traditions; sometimes they match, and at other times they are in sharp contrast. At some time, each of us is convinced that there is only one way to decide–my way! If social workers are unclear about or misunderstand the goal of medical treatment and the social work role, then the conflicts will most certainly be exacerbated. In order to help patients understand their options social workers need to clarify their own values and to respect the values of their colleagues, even when they differ. One of the benefits of working with cancer patients and their families is that social workers can usually do so over a period of time. It is the development of the relationships between the patient, physician, social worker, nurse, and other members of the team that encourages a respect for a variety of beliefs, thus helping everyone to negotiate the difficult ethical issues.

PEER SUPPORT

Another component in professional development is the importance of peer support. Having colleagues who immediately understand the work one does, without having to explain, contributes to a sense of professional satisfaction. Social workers who work in teaching hospitals or cancer centers may have easier access to such support, but there are options for those with less built-in support.

In many parts of the country, local or regional groups of oncology social workers meet regularly to provide ongoing education and support.

These groups are open to any social worker with an interest in oncology. The National Association of Oncology Social Workers (NAOSW) is an organization whose mission includes advocating sound public and professional programs and policies for cancer patients, creating professional standards for oncology social work practice, and providing valuable services to its members. NAOSW sponsors a yearly educational conference, publishes a quarterly newsletter, and offers consultation through its extensive network of members. Involvement with a local social work oncology group, as well as the national organization, guarantees access to a variety of learning experiences and other resources that are crucial to developing a sense of competence in this specialized area. For professionals acting as the sole oncology social worker in a particular setting, the peer support offered through these organizations can dramatically reduce the sense of isolation, in addition to providing excellent educational benefits.

CONTINUING EDUCATION

Rapidly changing treatment developments and the increased longevity of patients mandate the need for oncology social workers to continue to expand their knowledge and their repertoire of interventions, many of which have been discussed in other chapters of this resource book. It is not difficult to find programs and materials to meet a variety of continuing education needs, but in the current economic climate it is indeed difficult, if not impossible, for many social workers to be given time away from the workplace or financial assistance to take advantage of such offerings as seminars and courses. At the very least, social workers should be able to expect adequate and thorough orientation to their jobs. It is particularly helpful when your supervisor has specific oncology experience. Some new oncology social workers have been successful in obtaining outside specialized supervision when it is not available on site. The institution has a responsibility to provide support to staff and the social worker has the right to request supervision. This is an investment that pays off for the institution since it means not having to constantly replace inadequately trained, overwhelmed staff members who have been insufficiently prepared for their jobs.

The American Cancer Society, through its Division and Unit Professional Education Committees, provides a variety of educational programs at little or no cost to attendees. Many of the programs are scheduled at the end of the work day or on Saturdays in order to accommodate health professionals who cannot attend at other times.

MANAGING THE INTENSITY OF THE WORK

Oncology social workers frequently are asked to explain how they manage the intensity of their work over time. This query is generally followed by observations that the oncology social worker must either qualify for sainthood or find the work inordinately depressing. This is not a description that most social workers find useful, especially when new to the field of oncology. However, these well-intentioned comments do force staff to consider both the positive and negative impacts of the work. Identifying sources of stress and developing strategies to manage the physical and emotional aspects of the work are crucial to maintaining professional and personal balance.

During the 1970s and well into the 1980s, much was written about the burnout associated with the helping professions. Burnout has been a term frequently used to describe the long-term responses of persons on the front lines in social service agencies and health care settings. A more recent expression to describe this phenomenon is *compassion fatigue,* but the syndrome has not changed. It can occur when physical and psychological resources are depleted by the constant demand for a person's energy, expertise, and compassion. People are most vulnerable when they set unrealistically high expectations for themselves and for those with whom they work. Oncology social workers are prime candidates for compassion fatigue, especially when their empathy is not balanced by a flexible approach to the work and the ability to work toward their own goals, not those set by others.

The first step in developing a self-support protocol is to identify and validate what an individual finds difficult about the work and recognize that it is not useful to generalize; what is particularly distressing for one social worker may not be for another. It is precisely the variations in personality, prior experiences with illness and death, current life situation, training, supervision, and length of time in the field that determine what will create work-related stress for an individual.

It helps to learn early in clinical practice that there are limitations to what an individual social worker can accomplish and that setting both limits and realistic goals helps each member of the team, as well as patients and their families, maintain appropriate boundaries. One of the pitfalls for social workers new to the field is a sense of urgency about helping patients. When this translates into "doing for" patients rather than helping patients do for themselves, workers run the risk of removing even more control from patients and overextending themselves in unhealthy and unprofessional ways.

It is not enough to focus on what is difficult about the work. It is equally important to discover what counterbalances the sadness, frustration, and fatigue that inevitably occur. Social workers need to develop supportive networks inside as well as outside of the workplace and to create strategies that consistently nurture and replenish. It is important to find ways to divert attention from the intensity of ongoing interactions with patients and families. By evaluating their own coping strategies and substituting more adaptive ones for those that are less effective, social workers can substantially reduce their vulnerability.

Much has been written about the parallel process involved in oncology work. When the issues faced by patients and their families and their coping mechanisms are examined, it becomes clear that social workers and other members of the health care team experience the same feelings of uncertainty, denial, and the need to sustain hope that characterize the cancer experience. This parallel process has an effect on relationships. Just as it affects the balance within the family, it affects the balance of the team. Understanding this process can help social workers develop their role on the team.

Recognition of the value of the other members of the health care team contributes to a sense of shared responsibility and can significantly reduce the unwelcome sense of uniqueness that occurs when a person works in relative isolation. Such recognition is not always easy, especially in settings where competition among staff members produces excessive tension. Social workers often play a significant role in enhancing team cohesiveness. Quite frequently, they are expected to assume the role of team leader and conflict mediator. Although not always explicitly stated, social workers are viewed as having the skills necessary to bring the team together. Such leadership has enormous value in settings where the stress is inordinately high, especially when the social worker facilitates mutual respect among the individual members of the team.

COPING STRATEGIES

This section is not intended to provide a list of every adaptive coping strategy used by social workers in cancer care; however, a few should be highlighted.

In addition to achieving a skill level at which social workers feel competent, understand what is difficult in the work, and learn to set priorities and limits, the worker new to oncology must also learn how to balance the commitment to the job with a satisfying life outside. Just as one cannot look directly at the sun for very long without turning away, oncology social workers must find ways to divert their attention from their work. As well, it helps to discover when to take brief and extended breaks from work. The more indispensable social workers allow themselves to feel on the job, the more difficult it becomes to take care of themselves in a healthy way. Staff members who are unable to let go of the job, even for a well-deserved day off or a vacation of reasonable length, may find themselves so depleted that the only recourse they see is to make a premature permanent job change.

Any discussion of coping would be incomplete without mentioning the effectiveness of humor. For some, this may be the most adaptive way to cope with the demands and stress of the work. In learning to take work, but not oneself, too seriously there is an opportunity to sit back and put things into perspective. Humor, in its best sense, can be viewed as an expression of caring, for oneself and for others. Like everything else in life, medical settings spawn their own unique brand of humor. Although hospital humor is not meant to be disrespectful, an outsider might consider some of the humor a bit macabre. It is important to remember that there are funny moments–even in cancer.

In order for social workers to be effective in this work, they must possess self-awareness. Learning to identify their own patterns of stress and evaluating typical responses for managing the stress helps them seek alternatives to less-adaptive responses. Learning when it is time to make a change is equally important.

RESEARCH

Social workers are participating in psychosocial oncology research more actively than ever before. The results of research studies are published in a variety of journals, such as the *Journal of Psychosocial Oncology.* Most of the research has come out of direct clinical experience.

This experience identified certain groups of patients as being at higher risk for requiring more social work services. Other ideas emerge simply out of the social worker's own interest. Once an idea is formed, the non-research social worker may wonder how to develop it into a research study. If a researcher is not available within your hospital or agency, many schools of social work have the capability and interest to assist a social worker in implementing the study and even in helping collect the data. Research that culminates in new interventions enhances practice and, not incidentally, the credibility of social work.

Most oncology social workers do not have research opportunities built into their job descriptions. Time constraints are very real, but the wealth of clinical experience that is accrued over time provides some excellent research opportunities. Small studies can be undertaken with a moderate degree of additional effort.

With the current emphasis on quality assurance, research is another way to refine, monitor, and evaluate practice while contributing knowledge to the field. Hospital and agency administrators can more easily be convinced of the value of allotting time and resources to research when they feel that the end results might benefit the institution fiscally or improve patient services.

The American Cancer Society funds research related to the psychosocial aspects of cancer. Information about grants can be obtained through its national office in Atlanta.

CHANGES IN THE HEALTH CARE SYSTEM

Changes in the delivery of health care across the country have significantly affected social work practice, both in hospitals and community agencies. Shorter hospital stays have shifted the focus from inpatient to outpatient care. At the same time that social workers are expected to maximize continuity of care for patients and coordinate community resources for them, communities are battling the financial constraints that prevent them from providing services. Even when community resources exist, the large number of people lacking adequate insurance coverage compounds an already difficult situation. This situation requires enormous creativity and perseverance on the part of social workers and tests their advocacy skills, as well. Social workers often find themselves promoting and even developing new community resources. Acting as a liaison with community agencies has become an essential component of practice. At times, the social worker's role is to help patients and families access whatever resources are available and to advocate for those that are clearly needed, but do not yet exist. Patients, encouraged to become activists, often gain a sense of mastery in advocating, not only for themselves, but for others with similar needs.

Since so much care is now being given outside of the hospital, there is a need for community-based professionals to have some education about cancer, its treatment, and its impact on the family. Many community professionals are reluctant to accept cancer patients because they lack basic information, do not know what to expect, and question their ability to manage their own reactions. The social worker who is familiar with cancer is in an excellent position to act as a resource to community agencies and schools.

INFLUENCING POLICY DEVELOPMENT

As social workers committed to the needs and rights of cancer patients and their families, it is easy to become immersed in direct service without considering that there is a role for individual workers and their professional organizations in the political sphere. A number of organizations are involved in advocacy for cancer patients. The American Cancer Society not only stays abreast of current issues affecting this population, but publishes up-to-date information on pending legislation, some of which it has initiated. The National Coalition for Cancer Survivorship also actively works to change the situation regarding issues such as discrimination, employability, and insurability for cancer survivors. The National Association of Oncology Social Workers (NAOSW) and the Association of Pediatric Oncology Social Workers (APOSW), with their steadily increasing memberships, have the potential to become powerful political voices for the rights of cancer patients. Through the efforts of these organizations, it is relatively easy for any social worker to learn about current issues and legislation affecting all cancer patients, as well as learn how to become involved as an individual and as a member of a growing constituency with the potential to be a strong lobbying force.

Every social worker, once adequately informed about the issues, can participate in the process. Writing to legislators urging support for specific bills is an effective yet relatively easy way to get involved. This activity can be extremely empowering, as it enhances professional credibility. Just as patients achieve a sense of mastery and control of their situation, professionals who care for them may benefit from becoming advocates. Political activism regarding cancer-related issues might also be considered another coping strategy and it is consistent with the role of the social worker as an agent of change.

SUMMARY

Oncology social work has established itself as a vital speciality in the psychosocial care of the cancer patient. Initially, oncology social workers found themselves caring for patients whose life expectancy was measured, at most, in months. Today, the focus is increasingly on survival and long-term effects of treatment, while still attending to the needs of patients who are in a terminal phase. The systems that care for patients have become intensely complex, placing new demands on everyone involved. Social work has responded by developing a highly respected speciality in oncology and by working collaboratively with other disciplines to bring a broad range of practice skills and innovative approaches to the provision of mental health services for cancer patients and their families. The professional issues are both numerous and complex. At times, it seems that more questions are raised than are answered, especially in the rapidly changing health care climate. Social workers are intrinsically involved, however, and are in a unique position to affect, directly and indirectly, the care of patients and their families.

RESOURCES IN CANCER CARE FOR ADULTS AND CHILDREN

Paula R. Fogelberg, MSW, LCSW
Julia H. Gaskell, MSW, MPH

Because of the complexity and chronicity of cancer, patients and their families can be expected to require a variety of supports as they move through the illness experience. Social workers not only are expected to be knowledgeable about existing resources, but also are expected to help patients and families access them. It is important to remember that many individuals may be uncomfortable with the notion of relying on outside supports. Social workers are in a unique position to help patients make the best use of those resources that support optimal family stability.

Social workers also provide valuable education to community agencies about the needs of families facing cancer. Patients now spend less time in acute care settings, creating a need for community-based agencies to be well prepared to meet increased demands for services. This trend makes it more imperative that social workers in all settings must be aware of resources for their clients.

What follows is a list of resources that should offer the reader enough initial information to pursue more specific sources of help. The list is not exhaustive, but represents organizations with a major commitment to cancer patients and their families.

This chapter is organized into the following categories:

- For Further Information About Cancer
- Treatment Locations
- Specific Cancer Information Sources
- Support Organizations
- Practical Assistance
- Home Care

- National Organizations for Patient Housing
- Transportation
- Wish Organizations
- Professional Organizations
- Education and Training

Resources specific to children are denoted by an asterisk (*).

FOR FURTHER INFORMATION ABOUT CANCER

American Cancer Society

National Office
1599 Clifton Road NE, Atlanta, GA 30329
(404) 320-3333
1-800-ACS-2345

The American Cancer Society, dedicated to the control and eradication of cancer, is the largest voluntary health agency in the world. It is organized primarily on a geographic basis with 58 incorporated chartered Divisions, usually states, and Local Units, usually organized by county. Programs are implemented and services provided through the local offices.

The Society is a basic resource for information about cancer and its treatment. Printed and audio-visual materials are available to the public; professional education publications are also provided. The toll-free number is maintained to handle questions and concerns about cancer.

Regional, State, and Local Units may provide patient and family education, information and guidance programs, in-hospital information centers, home care item loans, transportation services, employment/insurability information, and support and self-help groups. For specific programs, see listings under "Support Services."

State or Division Offices

American Cancer Society
Alabama Division, Inc.
504 Brookwood Blvd.
Birmingham, AL 35209
(205) 879-2242

American Cancer Society
Alaska Division, Inc.
406 W Fireweed Lane
Suite 204
Anchorage, AK 99503
(907) 277-8696

American Cancer Society
Arizona Division, Inc.
2929 Thomas Road
Phoenix, AZ 85016
(602) 224-0524

American Cancer Society
Arkansas Division, Inc.
901 N University
Little Rock, AR 72207
(501) 664-3480

American Cancer Society
California Division, Inc.
1710 Webster St.
Suite 210
Oakland, CA 94612
(510) 893-7900

American Cancer Society
Colorado Division, Inc.
2255 S Oneida
Denver, CO 80224
(303) 758-2030

American Cancer Society
Connecticut Division, Inc.
Barnes Park South
14 Village Lane
Wallingford, CT 06492
(203) 265-7161

American Cancer Society
Delaware Division, Inc.
92 Read's Way
Suite 205
New Castle, DE 19720
(302) 324-4227

American Cancer Society
District of Columbia Div., Inc.
1875 Connecticut Ave.
Suite 730
Washington, DC 20009
(202) 483-2600

American Cancer Society
Florida Division, Inc.
1001 S MacDill Ave.
Tampa, FL 33629
(813) 253-0541

American Cancer Society
Georgia Division, Inc.
46 Fifth St. NE
Atlanta, GA 30308
(404) 892-0026

American Cancer Society
Hawaii-Pacific Division, Inc.
200 North Vineyard Blvd.
Suite 100-A
Honolulu, HI 96817
(808) 531-1662

American Cancer Society
Idaho Division, Inc.
2676 Vista Ave.
Boise, ID 83705
(208) 343-4609

American Cancer Society
Illinois Division, Inc.
77 E Monroe
Floor 13
Chicago, IL 60603
(312) 641-6150

American Cancer Society
Indiana Division, Inc.
8730 Commerce Park Place
Indianapolis, IN 46268
(317) 872-4432

American Cancer Society
Iowa Division, Inc.
8364 Hickman Road
Suite D
West Des Moines, IA 50325
(515) 253-0147

American Cancer Society
Kansas Division, Inc.
1315 SW Arrowhead Road
Topeka, KS 66604
(913) 273-4114
(913) 273-4422

American Cancer Society
Kentucky Division, Inc.
701 W Muhammed Ali Blvd.
Louisville, KY 40201-1807
(502) 584-6782

American Cancer Society
Long Island Division, Inc.
145 Pidgeon Hill Road
Huntington Station, NY 11746
(516) 385-9100

American Cancer Society
Louisiana Division, Inc.
Fidelity Homestead Building
837 Gravier St.
Suite 700
New Orleans, LA 70112-1509
(504) 523-2029

American Cancer Society
Maine Division, Inc.
52 Federal St.
Brunswick, ME 04011
(207) 729-3339

American Cancer Society
Maryland Division, Inc.
8219 Town Center Dr.
Baltimore, MD 21236
(410) 931-6868

American Cancer Society
Massachusetts Division, Inc.
Carhart Memorial Building
247 Commonwealth Ave.
Boston, MA 02116
(617) 267-2650

American Cancer Society
Michigan Division, Inc.
1205 E Saginaw St.
Lansing, MI 48906
(517) 371-2920

American Cancer Society
Minnesota Division, Inc.
3316 W 66th St.
Minneapolis, MN 55435
(612) 925-2772

American Cancer Society
Mississippi Division, Inc.
1380 Livingstone Lane
Jackson, MS 39213
(601) 362-8874

American Cancer Society
Missouri Division, Inc.
3322 American Ave.
Jefferson City, MO 65102
(314) 893-4800

American Cancer Society
Montana Division, Inc.
17 N 26th St.
Billings, MT 59101
(406) 252-7111

American Cancer Society
Nebraska Division, Inc.
8502 West Center Road
Omaha, NE 68124-5255
(402) 393-5800

American Cancer Society
Nevada Division, Inc.
1325 E Harmon
Las Vegas, NV 89119
(702) 798-6857

American Cancer Society
New Hampshire Division, Inc.
360 Route 101 Unit 501
Bedford, NH 03110-5032
1-800-640-7101
(603) 472-8899

American Cancer Society
New Jersey Division, Inc.
2600 US Highway
North Brunswick, NJ
08902-0803
(908) 297-8000

American Cancer Society
New Mexico Division, Inc.
5800 Lomas Blvd. NE
Albuquerque, NM 87110
(505) 260-2105

American Cancer Society
New York City Division, Inc.
19 W 56th St.
New York, NY 10019
(212) 586-8700

American Cancer Society
New York State Division, Inc.
6725 Lyons St.
East Syracuse, NY 13057
(315) 437-7025

American Cancer Society
North Carolina Division, Inc.
11 S Boylan Ave.
Suite 221
Raleigh, NC 27603
(919) 834-8463

American Cancer Society
North Dakota Division, Inc.
123 Roberts St.
Fargo, ND 58102
(701) 232-1385

American Cancer Society
Ohio Division, Inc.
5555 Frantz Road
Dublin, OH 43017
(614) 889-9565

American Cancer Society
Oklahoma Division, Inc.
3000 United Founders Blvd.
Suite 136
Oklahoma City, OK 73112
(405) 843-9888

American Cancer Society
Oregon Division, Inc.
0330 SW Curry St.
Portland, OR 97201
(503) 295-6422

American Cancer Society
Pennsylvania Division, Inc.
Route 422 & Sipe Ave.
Hershey, PA 17033
(717) 533-6144

American Cancer Society
Philadelphia Division, Inc.
1422 Chestnut St.
2nd Floor
Philadelphia, PA 19102
(215) 665-2900

American Cancer Society
Puerto Rico Division, Inc.
Calle Alverio #577
Esquina Sargento Medina
Hato Rey, PR 00918
(809) 764-2295

American Cancer Society
Queens Division, Inc.
112-25 Queens Blvd.
Forest Hills, NY 11375
(718) 263-2224

American Cancer Society
Rhode Island Division, Inc.
400 Main St.
Pawtucket, RI 02860
(401) 722-8480

American Cancer Society
South Carolina Division, Inc.
128 Stonemark Lane
Westpark Plaza
Columbia, SC 29210
(803) 750-1693

American Cancer Society
South Dakota Division, Inc.
4101 Carnegie Place
Sioux Falls, SD 57106
(605) 361-8277

American Cancer Society
Tennessee Division, Inc.
1315 8th Ave. South
Nashville, TN 37203
(615) 255-1227

American Cancer Society
Texas Division, Inc.
2433 Ridgepoint Dr.
Austin, TX 78754
(512) 928-2262

American Cancer Society
Utah Division, Inc.
941 East 3300 South
Salt Lake City, UT 84102
(801) 483-1500

American Cancer Society
Vermont Division, Inc.
13 Loomis St.
Montpelier, VT 05602
(802) 223-2348

American Cancer Society
Virginia Division, Inc.
4240 Park Place Court
Glen Allen, VA 23060
(804) 527-3700

American Cancer Society
Washington Division, Inc.
2120 1st Ave. North
Seattle, WA 98109-1140
(206) 283-1152

American Cancer Society
Westchester Division, Inc.
30 Glenn St.
White Plains, NY 10603
(914) 949-4800

American Cancer Society
West Virginia Division, Inc.
2428 Kanawha Blvd. E
Charleston, WV 25311
(304) 344-3611

American Cancer Society
Wisconsin Division, Inc.
615 N Sherman Ave.
Madison, WI 53704
(608) 249-0487

American Cancer Society
Wyoming Division, Inc.
2222 House Ave.
Cheyenne, WY 82001
(307) 638-3331

*** ASSOCIATION FOR THE CARE OF CHILDREN'S HEALTH (ACCH)**

7910 Woodmont Ave., Suite 300, Bethesda, MD 20814
(301) 654-6549

A nonprofit, multidisciplinary organization of both health professionals and parents. Its aim is to promote psychosocial health and well being of children and their families in health care settings. It publishes a quarterly journal and two newsletters. ACCH also provides at a minimal cost a vast array of materials relating to the psychosocial aspects of children and health.

CANCER INFORMATION SERVICE
1-800-4-CANCER
Cancer Information Service (CIS) offices serve the entire United States to answer cancer-related questions from the general public, cancer patients and their families, and health professionals. Personnel at each CIS office are trained to provide accurate and easily understood information in response to each caller's cancer questions. There is no charge for the call or for the information provided.

Based on area code, callers are automatically routed to the CIS office serving their area. Approximately 80% of the U. S. population live in areas served by regional offices, including 31 states and metropolitan New York City. An office at the National Cancer Institute (NCI) serves the remainder of the country.

Health professionals can order from a range of free publications designed for their use. They can also order the lay language publications for distribution to patients and for their use in waiting rooms.

Source material used to respond to callers' questions is updated regularly by the NCI. A computerized database provides information on state-of-the art cancer treatment and current clinical research.

For free copies of the NCI Publications List for the Public and Patients and the NCI Publications List for Health Professionals, call: 1-800-4-CANCER* (1-800-422-6237).

Direct written requests to: The National Cancer Institute, Building 3 -Room 10A24, 9000 Rockville Pike, Bethesda, MD 20892-3100.

* In Alaska call 1-800-638-1234. Spanish-speaking staff members are available to callers in some areas.

*** CANCER ANSWER LINE**
1-800-ACS-2345
The American Cancer Society Cancer Answer Line provides answers to cancer-related questions from the general public, cancer patients and their families, and health professionals.

*** FEDERATION FOR CHILDREN WITH SPECIAL NEEDS**
95 Berkeley St., Suite 104, Boston, MA 02116
(617) 482-2915

A center for parents and parent organizations serving children and families.

* NATIONAL INFORMATION CENTER FOR HANDICAPPED CHILDREN AND YOUTH (NICHCY)

Box 1492, Washington, DC 20013
(703) 893-6061

Produces publications that meet general information and resource needs on rare disorders, chronic health problems.

PHYSICIAN DATA QUERY (PDQ)
1-800-4-CANCER
THE NATIONAL CANCER INSTITUTE'S COMPUTERIZED DATABASE FOR PHYSICIANS

PDQ (Physician Data Query) is a computer database for retrieval of cancer treatment information. PDQ's database has three major files: (1) summary of the most current approaches to cancer treatment; (2) research treatment protocols that are open to patient entry; (3) directory of physicians that provide cancer treatment and health care organizations that have programs of cancer care.

The cancer information file contains prognostic and treatment information on all major cancers. Each section includes a summary of state-of-the-art treatment that provides up-to-date information on prognosis, relevant staging and cellular classification systems, and listings of appropriate treatment options according to the type and stage of cancer.

The protocol file currently contains information on more than 1000 active clinical trials. It contains summaries of all the treatment protocols directly supported by NCI, as well as protocols that have been voluntarily submitted by other clinical investigators for inclusion in the PDQ system.

The staff of NCI's Cancer Information Service network (toll-free phone number is 1-800-4-CANCER) will provide a one-time-only service for physicians. At that time, physicians will be informed of other alternatives for obtaining information from PDQ (e.g., nearest medical library, National Library of Medicine [NLM], other vendors).

Medical libraries at medical centers that subscribe to the NLM service will also be able to access the full PDQ system. Currently, PDQ is accessible at over 8000 medical libraries and health care institutions throughout the United States.

TREATMENT LOCATIONS

The organizations listed can be used to identify accredited treatment centers.

Comprehensive and Clinical Cancer Centers Supported by the National Cancer Institute

The National Cancer Institute (NCI) supports a number of cancer centers throughout the country that develop and investigate new methods of cancer diagnosis and treatment. Information about referral procedures, treatment costs, and services available to patients can be obtained from the individual cancer centers listed below.

Alabama

University of Alabama Comprehensive Cancer Center
Basic Health Sciences Bldg., Room 108
1918 University Blvd., Birmingham, AL 35294-3300
(205) 934-6612/(205) 934-5077

Arizona

University of Arizona Cancer Center
1501 N Campbell Ave., Tucson, AZ 85724
(602) 626-6372

California

The Kenneth Norris Jr. Comprehensive Cancer Center and
The Kenneth Norris Jr. Hospital Research Institute
University of Southern California
1441 Eastlake Ave., Los Angeles, CA 90033-0804
(213) 226-2370

Jonsson Comprehensive Cancer Center (UCLA)
200 Medical Plaza, Suite 120, Los Angeles, CA 90027
(213) 206-0278

City of Hope National Medical Center
Beckman Research Institute
1500 E Duarte Road, Duarte, CA 91010
(818) 359-8111

University of California at San Diego Cancer Center
225 Dickinson St., San Diego, CA 92103-8421
(619) 543-6178

Colorado
University of Colorado Cancer Center
4200 E 9th Ave., Box B190, Denver, CO 80262
(303) 270-7235

Connecticut
Yale University Comprehensive Cancer Center
333 Cedar St., New Haven, CT 06510
(203) 785-6338

District of Columbia
Lombardi Cancer Research Center
Georgetown University Medical Center
3800 Reservoir Road NW, Washington, DC 20007
(202) 687-2192

Florida
Sylvester Comprehensive Cancer Center
University of Miami Medical School
1475 NW 12th Ave., Miami, FL 33136
(305) 548-4800

Illinois
Illinois Cancer Council (Consortium)
17th Floor, 200 S Michigan Ave., Chicago, IL 60604
(312) 986-9980

University of Chicago Cancer Research Center
5841 S Maryland Ave., Chicago, IL 60637
(312) 702-9200

Kentucky
Lucille Parker Markey Cancer Center
University of Kentucky Medical Center
800 Rose St., Lexington, KY 40536-0093
(606) 257-4447

Maryland
The Johns Hopkins Oncology Center
600 N Wolfe St., Baltimore, MD 21205
(301) 955-8638

Massachusetts
Dana-Farber Cancer Institute
44 Binney St., Boston, MA 02115
(617) 632-3000

Michigan
Meyer L. Prentis Comprehensive Cancer Center
of Metropolitan Detroit
110 E Warren Ave., Detroit, MI 48201
(313) 936-2516

Minnesota
Mayo Comprehensive Cancer Center
200 1st St. SW, Rochester, MN 55905
(507) 284-3322

New Hampshire
Norris Cotton Cancer Center
Dartmouth-Hitchcock Medical Center
2 Maynard St., Hanover, NH 03756
(603) 646-5505

New York
Memorial Sloan-Kettering Cancer Center
1275 York Ave., New York, NY 10021
1-800-525-2225

Columbia University Cancer Center
College of Physicians and Surgeons
630 W 168th St., New York, NY 10032
(212) 305-8081

North Carolina
Duke Comprehensive Cancer Center
P.O. Box 3814, Durham, NC 27710
(919) 286-5515

Lineberger Comprehensive Cancer Center
University of North Carolina School of Medicine
Chapel Hill, NC 27599
(919) 966-4431

Cancer Center of Wake Forest University at the
Bowman Gray School of Medicine
300 S Hawthorne Road, Winston-Salem, NC 27103
(919) 748-4354

Ohio
Ohio State University Comprehensive Cancer Center
410 W 10th Ave., Columbus, OH 43210
(614) 293-8619

Case Western Reserve University
University Hospitals of Cleveland, Ireland Cancer Center
2074 Abington Road, Cleveland, OH 44106
(216) 844-5432

Pennsylvania
Fox Chase Cancer Center
7701 Burholme Ave., Philadelphia, PA 19111
(215) 728-6900

University of Pennsylvania Cancer Center
3400 Civic Center Bldg., Philadelphia, PA 19104
(215) 662-6364

Pittsburgh Cancer Institute
369 Victoria Bldg., Pittsburgh, PA 15261
1-800-537-4063

Rhode Island
Roger Williams Medical Center
825 Chalkstone Ave., Providence, RI 02908
(401) 456-2070

Tennessee
St. Jude Children's Research Hospital
332 N Lauderdale, Memphis, TN 38105
(901) 522-0694

Texas
The University of Texas M. D. Anderson Cancer Center
1515 Holcombe Blvd., Houston, TX 77030
(713) 792-6161

Utah
Utah Regional Cancer Center
University of Utah Medical Center
50 North Medical Dr., Room 2C 110, Salt Lake City, UT 84132
(801) 581-4048

Vermont
Vermont Regional Cancer Center
University of Vermont
1 S Prospect St., Burlington, VT 05401
(802) 656-4580

Virginia
Medical College of Virginia, Massey Cancer Center
401 College St., Richmond, VA 23298
(804) 786 0450

University of Virginia Medical Center
P.O. Box 334, Charlottesville, VA 22908
(804) 924-2562

Washington
Fred Hutchinson Cancer Research Center
1124 Columbia St., Seattle, WA 98104
(206) 467-4675

Wisconsin
Wisconsin Clinical Cancer Center
University of Wisconsin
600 Highland Ave., Madison, WI 53792
(608) 263-8090

AMERICAN COLLEGE OF SURGEONS

55 E Erie, Chicago, IL 60611-9976
(312) 664-4050

The Commission on Cancer of the American College of Surgeons has as its primary objective improving the quality of care for patients with cancer. One of its committees is responsible for reviewing and approving cancer programs in hospitals that request a survey on a voluntary basis.

A listing of hospitals having approved cancer programs can be obtained from this office.

ASSOCIATION OF COMMUNITY CANCER CENTERS

11600 Nebel Street, Suite 201, Rockville, MD 20852
(301) 984-9496

Provides a mechanism for the exchange of information among health professionals who believe high-quality cancer care should be available in the community. Publishes *Community Cancer Centers* in the United States and *The Journal of Cancer Program Management.*

INTERNATIONAL UNION AGAINST CANCER

(Union Internationale Center Le Cancer–UICC)
3 rue du conseil–General
1205 Geneva, Switzerland
41-22 20 18-11

Nongovernmental, voluntary organization devoted to worldwide campaign against cancer in its research, therapeutic, and preventive aspects.

Exchange of information is facilitated between national cancer organizations. Publishes, with NCI support, *International Directory of Specialized Cancer Research and Treatment Establishments.*

SPECIFIC CANCER INFORMATION SOURCES

ASSOCIATION FOR BRAIN TUMOR RESEARCH

3725 N Talman Ave., Chicago, IL 60618
(312) 286-5571

Voluntary organization that supports research, promotes the understanding of brain tumors, and offers printed materials that deal with research and treatment of brain tumors.

* CHILDREN'S LEUKEMIA FOUNDATION OF MICHIGAN

19022 W Ten Mile Road, Southfield, MI 48075-2498
1-800-825-2536/(313) 353-8222

Provides financial aid for Michigan residents with blood-related disorders. Publishes *Friends Helping Friends: Bone Marrow Transplant Resource Guide,* which gives practical information including tips about fundraising and a listing of resources for bone marrow transplant patients.

HYSTERECTOMY EDUCATIONAL RESOURCES AND SERVICES

422 Bryn Mawr Ave., Bala Cynwyd, PA 19004
(215) 667-7757

Furnishes information by phone and provides counseling for women prior to surgery and after surgery. Lending library, newsletter, and second opinion information available.

INTERNATIONAL ASSOCIATION OF LARYNGECTOMEES (IAL)

Contact the Local Unit of the American Cancer Society for services in area.

Provides information and supportive materials to laryngectomee patients, as well as pre- and postoperative support from laryngectomee volunteers. Promotes and supports rehabilitation programs.

LEUKEMIA SOCIETY OF AMERICA, INC.

National Office, 733 3rd Ave., New York, NY 10017
(212) 573-8484

A voluntary health agency dedicated to meeting the special needs of people with leukemia, lymphoma, and multiple myeloma. The Society provides detailed information on those illnesses and offers a broad range of programs including financial aid, support groups for patients and families, and other means of local assistance.

The society also conducts a full-scale public and professional awareness and education program throughout the United States and, since its foundation in 1949, has sponsored over $60 million in research into the causes and cures of leukemia and related diseases.

For further information, contact the Society's national headquarters (address and telephone number shown) or one of the chapter offices located in the following states and cities. For local address and telephone number refer to your telephone directory.

Alabama
Birmingham

Arizona
Phoenix

California
Los Angeles
Sacramento
San Diego
San Francisco
Tustin
(Orange County)

Colorado
Denver

Connecticut
Darien
Hamden
Hartford

Delaware
Wilmington

Dist. of Columbia
Alexandria, VA

Florida
Jacksonville
Miami
Orlando
Tampa
West Palm Beach

Georgia
Atlanta

Illinois
Chicago

Indiana
Indianapolis

Kansas
Wichita

Kentucky
Louisville

Louisiana
New Orleans

Maryland
Baltimore

Massachusetts
Boston

Michigan
Detroit

Minnesota
Minneapolis

Missouri
Kansas City
St. Louis

New Jersey
Lindenwood
Maplewood

New York
Albany
Buffalo
Hicksville
New York City
Rochester
Syracuse
White Plains

North Carolina
Charlotte

Ohio
Cincinnati
Cleveland
Columbus

Oklahoma
Oklahoma City

Oregon
Portland

Pennsylvania
Harrisburg
Philadelphia
Pittsburgh

Rhode Island
Cranston

South Carolina
Columbia

Tennessee
Nashville

Texas
Dallas/Ft.Worth
Houston
San Antonio

Virginia
Hampton

Washington
Seattle

Wisconsin
Milwaukee

The following lists leukemia informational materials available. Contact Leukemia Society of America, local chapter.

Literature
Facts About the Leukemia Society of America
Leukemia
Lymphomas
Hodgkin's Disease
Multiple Myeloma
Research
Patient-Aid Program
What Everyone Should Know About Leukemia
Leukemia–The Nature of the Disease
Leukemia Quiz
Facts About Leukemia and Related Diseases (Blue Leaflet)
Emotional Aspects of Childhood Leukemia
Bone Marrow Transplantation
What It Is That I Have, Don't Want, etc. (Teen Diary)
Acute Myelogenous Leukemia
Chronic Myelogenous Leukemia
Acute Lymphocytic Leukemia
Chronic Lymphocytic Leukemia
Understanding Chemotherapy

Learn About Leukemia–A Coloring and Activity Book
Making Intelligent Choices About Therapy
Family Support Group
Coping With Survival
I'm Having a Bone Marrow Transplant (Coloring Book)
Someone Likes You Beary Much (Limited Supply–Activity Book for Siblings)

Video/Films
A Sense of Hope (13 min: Joey, young leukemia patient)
You're Not Alone (26 min: leukemia patient experiences/support)
Must Win (15/26 min: Gary Carter, New York Mets)
What It Is That I Have, Don't Want, etc. (24 min: Teens)
A Critical Decision (17 min: bone marrow transplants)
Otteau Christiansen "Victory Story" (16 min: bone marrow patient)
Jansen-Beres Story (10 min: Olympic speedskater)
Closing In On A Cure (20 min: Otteau Christiansen-facts update)

Update and Reprints
Facts About Leukemia–6 page report on the disease prepared by LSA staff
Radiation and Nuclear Power–6 page report by Kenneth McCredie, MD
Cat Leukemia: Research Into its Origins Hold Promise for Man – 7 page report/Q&A
Thirty Years of Progress: The Story of the Leukemia Society (12 page history)
1989 Research Report–5 page report by Peter Quesenberry, MD
Interleukin-2 and Society Research–2 page report
Interferon and Hairy Cell Leukemia–4 page report
Aids and Leukemia Research

NATIONAL AIDS HOTLINE

(800) 342-2437 (24 hours)
(800) 344-7432 Spanish-speaking (8:00 A.M. to 2:00 A.M.)
(800) 243-7889 hearing-impaired (8:00 A.M. to 10:00 P.M.)

NATIONAL ALLIANCE OF BREAST CANCER ORGANIZATIONS (NABCO)

1180 Avenue of the Americas, Second Floor
New York, NY 10036
(212) 719-0154

Established to provide unity among organizations and individuals in the fight against breast cancer and to serve as a resource for persons who have concerns about breast cancer and other breast diseases. NABCO also seeks to have an impact on public and private policy in the areas of insurance reimbursements, funding priorities, and health legislation dealing with breast cancer at the national, state, and local levels.

THE NATIONAL BONE MARROW DONOR PROGRAM

c/o Director of Operations
3433 Broadway St. NW, Suite 400, Minneapolis, MN 55413
1-800-654-1247

A collaborative effort of the American Association of Blood Banks, the National American Red Cross, and the Council of Community Blood Centers. (Formerly the National Bone Marrow Donor Registry.) It offers information on being a donor or locating a donor for bone marrow transplantation.

THE ORGAN TRANSPLANT FUND

1027 S Yates, Memphis, TN 38119
(901) 684-1697

Helps patients raise and delegate funds for organ transplants, including bone marrow transplants, and transplant-related expenses. Maintains accounts to which tax-deductible contributions can be made on the transplant patient's behalf.

*THE CHILDREN'S ORGAN TRANSPLANT ASSOCIATION (COTA)

917 S Rogers St., Bloomington, IN 47403
1-800-366-2682/(812) 336-8872

COTA assists families with children in need of an organ transplant, including bone marrow transplant, organize fundraisers in their communities.

*CHILDREN'S TRANSPLANT ASSOCIATION

P.O. Box 53699, Dallas, TX 75253
(214) 287-8484

Provides counseling and financial assistance to patients (both adults and children) in need of solid organ or bone marrow transplants.

THE NIELSEN TRANSPLANT FOUNDATION

580 W 8th St., Jacksonville, FL 32209

Provides aid to Northeast Florida residents in need of organ transplants. Educates people in need of a transplant, helps establish bank accounts for donations, assists patients in finding avenues of funding, and pays for certain aspects of transplants not covered by insurance.

***Some states have special programs (other than Medicaid) to assist children needing bone marrow transplants. In California, call California Children's Services, (916) 322-2090. In Florida, call Children's Medical Services, (904) 488-5040. In Michigan, call Children's Special Health Care Services, (517) 335-8961. In other states, call your state Department of Health to find out if a transplant assistance program exists.**

UNITED OSTOMY ASSOCIATION

36 Executive Park, Suite 120, Irvine, CA 92714
(714) 660-8624

A nonprofit organization that provides speakers, literature, and monthly information meetings for people who have a colostomy, ileostomy, or urostomy. Volunteers, most of whom are ostomates, may visit patients with ostomies in the hospital or home with the consent of the patients' physicians. The organization publishes a magazine, *Ostomy Quarterly,* and has publications and slide programs on every aspect of ostomies.

Y-ME NATIONAL ORGANIZATION FOR BREAST CANCER INFORMATION AND SUPPORT

18220 Harwood Ave., Homewood, IL 60430
(708) 799-8228 (Business Phone)
(Patient Hotline) 1-800-221-2141 (Outside 708 area code)
(Patient Hotline) 799-8228 (Inside 708 area code)

Provides information and peer support to breast cancer patients via Hotline and monthly education meetings. Provides workshops to professionals on psychosocial aspects of breast cancer. Publishes a newsletter.

SUPPORT ORGANIZATIONS

AMERICAN CANCER SOCIETY

Although services for cancer patients and their families vary throughout the country, each unit is expected to develop and maintain a minimum, or basic, patient services program consisting of:

- *Resources, information, and guidance.* Specific information on cancer and its treatment is provided as well as information on community resources and American Cancer Society services. The Society provides information about employability rights to individuals who have received a diagnosis of cancer and about insurability issues. Many Divisions and Units are involved in advocacy efforts for persons with cancer health histories who are experiencing employability or insurability problems.

- *Home care.* This service provides cancer patients with dressings, home care supplies, gift items for care and comfort, and information and education regarding home care practices. In addition, durable medical equipment can be loaned or rented for use in the patient's home.

- *Rehabilitation programs.* A number of programs are available to assist cancer patients to function at normal or near normal capacity and to resume their place in the family, community, and workplace. This service provides patient and family assistance in understanding the disease and its management through group education and mutual aid programs and the provision of pamphlets, booklets, and audio-visual presentations.

Patient Visitor Programs

These services are provided by carefully selected and trained visitors who have successfully managed the cancer experience.

REACH TO RECOVERY

This program is designed to assist the woman who has or has had breast cancer to meet the physical, emotional, and cosmetic needs related to her disease and its treatment.

OSTOMY

This program is designed to provide emotional support and information to individuals with an ostomy due to intestinal or urinary cancers so they may function at an optimal physical and social level.

LARYNGECTOMY

This service is designed to promote and support the rehabilitation of an individual who has had surgical removal of the larynx (laryngectomy).

CANSURMOUNT OR CANSUPPORT

This is a visitor program that provides functional, emotional, and social support for patients with cancers other than those listed earlier, and for family members.

Group Programs

I CAN COPE

A structured group education course for patients and family members that provides information on cancer, its treatment, side effects, nutrition, body image and self-esteem, available resources, and other topics.

SUPPORT GROUPS, MUTUAL AID GROUPS

Most Units have as resources support groups conducted under the leadership of professionals and mutual aid or self-help groups conducted by trained lay volunteers.

LOOK GOOD, FEEL BETTER

A program developed by the Cosmetic, Toiletry and Fragrance Association (CTFA) Foundation, the National Cosmetology Association, and the American Cancer Society, specifically for cancer patients undergoing chemotherapy or radiation treatments. Tips for improving one's appearance are given in a brochure available through local American Cancer Society offices. Local American Cancer Society offices may also offer workshops conducted by a trained representative of the National Cosmetology Association.

Other Programs

Some Units provide additional programs such as:

HOUSING (GUESTROOM PROGRAM)

Many Divisions and Units secure free hotel/motel accommodations for patients who have to travel long distances from their homes for treatment. Application should be made to the Division that serves the location where treatment is to be provided.

HOME HEALTH CARE

Household assistance to patients may be available on a limited basis in some areas.

MEDICATIONS

Some Divisions provide financial support for the minimal cost of therapeutic and palliative drugs for medically indigent patients.

*** CHILDREN'S PROGRAMS**

A variety of services and programs are offered throughout the country, including oncology camps, recreational activities (both for children with cancer and for children of adult cancer patients), support groups, parents' groups, and schools.

*CAMPS FOR CHILDREN

***Children's Oncology Camps of America**
Children's Memorial Hospital
2300 Children's Plaza, Box 30, Chicago, IL 60614
Attn: Edward Baum, MD
(312) 880-4564

Provides up-to-date listing of camps for children with cancer, listed by state.

***Camp Simcha**
5323 12th Ave., Brooklyn, NY 11219
(914) 856-1432

Camp Simcha is the only Kosher camp in the world for children with cancer, aplastic anemia, and related diseases.

***Starlight Foundation International**
12233 W Olympic Blvd., Suite 322, Los Angeles, CA 90064
(213) 207-5558

***Sunshine Foundation of Florida**
P.O. Box 255, Loughman, FL 33858
1-800-457-1976

See also "Candlelighters Childhood Cancer Foundation"

CANCER FAMILY CARE

Central Office
7710 Reading Road, Suite 204, Cincinnati, OH 45237
(513) 821-3346

Northern Kentucky Office
11 Shelby St., Florence, KY 41042-1612
(606) 525-6829

Clermont County Office
2085A Front Wheel Dr., Batavia, OH 45103
(513) 724-6005

A United Appeal Agency offering counseling to cancer patients and their families in Hamilton, Brown, Clermont, and Warren Counties in Ohio; and in Boone, Kenton, and Campbell Counties in Northern Kentucky.

* CANDLELIGHTERS CHILDHOOD CANCER FOUNDATION

1312 18th St. NW, Suite 200, Washington, DC 20036
1-800-366-2223

Provides the coordination and educational arm of an international network of self-help groups. Provides publications, including quarterly newsletters for parents and teenagers, and an annotated bibliography and resource guide. In addition, Candlelighters provides the development of educational materials on pediatric cancer and the needs of patients and families. Foundation has a listing of camps for children and their siblings.

* CENTERING CORPORATION

1531 N Saddle Creek Road, Omaha, NE 68104
(402) 553-1200

Provides workshops, information, and resources on the hospitalized child and on caring for the family of the dying and deceased child.

*** CHAI LIFELINE**

48 W 25th St., 6th Floor, New York, NY 10010
(212) 255-1160

Provides a variety of programs and information for Jewish children with cancer.

*** COMPASSIONATE FRIENDS**

P.O. Box 3696, Oakbrook, IL 60522-3696
(708) 990-0010

A self-help organization with chapters in various locations nationwide offering friendship and support to bereaved parents. Publishes a newsletter and other materials on parent and sibling bereavement. National office is the coordinating arm for local chapters.

Check with local hospice organizations for other bereavement groups. See listing "National Hospice Organization."

CONCERN FOR DYING

250 W 57th St., New York, NY 10107
(212) 246-6962

Nonprofit educational council that advocates an individual's right to participate in decisions regarding his or her treatment, particularly those decisions when a person is near death. Services provided include: information regarding the living will and up-to-date information on the current laws of each state concerning euthanasia, death, and dying; psychological and legal counseling; and referral to local organizations for other types of assistance.

ENCORE

YWCA of the United States
726 Broadway, 5th Floor, New York, NY 10003
(212) 614-2827

Encore provides postmastectomy group and rehabilitation programs, including support groups and special water and floor exercises. Contact the YWCA in your area first to learn about a local Encore program. The national office of the YWCA trains staff, certifies each program, and can help you locate the nearest Encore program in your community.

MAKE TODAY COUNT

101 1/2 S Union St., Alexandria, VA 22314
(703) 548-9674

An international organization for persons with cancer or other life-threatening illnesses. Local chapters provide emotional self-help through formal programs, group discussions, newsletters, social activities, workshops and seminars, and educational activities.

NATIONAL AIDS HOTLINE

1-800-342-AIDS (Spanish speaking)
1-800-344-SIDA (Learning impaired)
1-800-AIDSTTY (Hearing impaired)

NATIONAL COALITION FOR CANCER SURVIVORSHIP (NCCS)

1010 Wayne Ave., Suite 300, Silver Spring, MD 20910
(301) 585-2616

A network of independent organizations and individuals working in the area of cancer support and survivorship. The primary goal is to generate a nationwide awareness of cancer survivorship. NCCS facilitates communications between persons involved with cancer survivorship, promotes the development of cancer support activities, advocates the interest of cancer survivors, and encourages the study of survivorship. NCCS edited a book entitled *Charting the Journey: An Almanac of Practical Resources for Cancer Survivors,* a Consumer Reports Book published by Consumers Union. A publications form for ordering this and other materials is available from the above address.

***SIBLING INFORMATION NETWORK**

A.J. Pappanikou Center
991 Main St., East Hartford, CT 06108
(203) 282-7050

Provides resources addressing needs of siblings of persons with disabilities and chronic illnesses. Quarterly newsletters are available by subscription.

TOUCH

513 Tinsley Harrison Tower, University Station
Birmingham, AL 35294
(205) 934-3814

TOUCH stands for "Today Our Understanding of Cancer is Hope." It is cosponsored by the American Cancer Society Alabama Division, Inc., and the Comprehensive Cancer Center, Birmingham, AL. There are several hundred members in a number of different cities in Alabama. The program offers emotional and psychological support to cancer patients who are undergoing or have completed cancer treatment, and their significant others.

Y-ME NATIONAL ORGANIZATION FOR BREAST CANCER INFORMATION AND SUPPORT

18220 Harwood Ave., Homewood, IL 60430
(708) 799-8228 (Business phone)
(Patient Hotline) 1-800-221-2141 (Outside 708 area code)
(Patient Hotline) 799-8228 (Inside 708 area code)

Provides information and peer support to breast cancer patients via Hotline and monthly education meetings. Provides workshops to professionals on psychosocial aspects of breast cancer. Publishes a newsletter.

PRACTICAL ASSISTANCE

AMERICAN ASSOCIATION OF RETIRED PERSONS (AARP)

601 E St. NW, Washington, DC 20049
(202) 434-227

Nonprofit organization open to persons 50 years of age and older for nominal membership fee. Of particular interest to cancer patients is the drug-buying service at reduced prices. Prescription drugs, vitamins, and drug products can be obtained by members through a mail order service.

AMERICAN CANCER SOCIETY

1-800-ACS-2345

Practical assistance for housing during treatment, transportation to and from treatment, loan and gift items, and minimal financial support for medically indigent may be provided. Services vary among local communities.

Restrictions
American Cancer Society funds cannot be used to pay bills for services rendered to cancer patients by hospitals, clinics, nursing homes, physicians, or other health care professionals. Such professional services include diagnostic and therapeutic radiology, surgery, chemotherapy, and other diagnostic or treatment activities. Many Divisions and Units have additional restrictions. Inquire locally.

CANCER CARE

1180 Avenue of the Americas, New York, NY 10036
(212) 221-3300

The service arm of the National Cancer Foundation, Cancer Care is a nonprofit social service agency dedicated to helping patients and families cope with the emotional, psychological, and financial consequences of cancer. Although the organization primarily serves New York City and its tri-state, metropolitan region, it also responds to letters and phone calls from all over the United States, providing information and referrals whenever possible.

CANCER FUND OF AMERICA

2901 Breezewood Lane, Knoxville, TN 37921
(615) 938-5281

Provides up to $75/month in aid to medically indigent cancer patients.

*CHILDREN'S SPECIAL HEALTH SERVICES (FORMERLY CRIPPLED CHILDREN)

Administered under the Department of Human Resources, the port of entry is usually the Public Health Department. Coverage and eligibility vary from state to state. Covers medical bills, drugs, and equipment.

COMPREHENSIVE HEALTH INSURANCE POOL (CHIP)

Contact specific State Department of Insurance.

Several states have adopted programs of health insurance to residents who are unable to find adequate health insurance coverage in the private market due to their mental or physical condition. Insurance may be purchased even though the individual is not insurable in other plans.

COBRA

Under Public Law 99-272 employers sponsoring group health plans must offer employees and their families a temporary extension of coverage in certain instance where coverage would otherwise end. People who would have lost their insurance coverage due to a change in work circumstances such as being laid off, fired, or through quitting, now may be provided continued group insurance coverage for 18 months (employees) or 36 months (spouses, dependents).

FINANCIAL RESOURCES

Medicaid provides insurance coverage for indigent and low-income families. Services are coordinated by local Departments of Social Services. Medicaid recipients may obtain assistance with transportation through their local Department of Social Services. See "Social Security" section for further information.

Public assistance and other government-supported resources available for families dealing with illness are not to be forgotten or overlooked when dealing with a cancer diagnosis. Such resources would include:

- Children's Special Health Services (formerly Crippled Children's Services)
- Department of Human Services –Family Assistance including Aid to Families with Dependent Children, Food Stamps, and medically needy
- Vocational Rehabilitation
- Veterans Administration

HILL BURTON ACT–US PUBLIC HEALTH SERVICE

1-800-638-0742

Some hospitals who received monies under the Hill Burton Act are required to provide some indigent care. A recorded answering service at the above number gives information on Hill Burton hospitals. Information can be sent on these hospitals.

LEUKEMIA RESEARCH FOUNDATION

899 Skokie Blvd., Northbrook, IL 60062
(708) 480-1177
Pays up to $1500 per leukemia patient (both children and adults) over a

period of two years to assist with medical expenses.

SOCIAL SECURITY ADMINISTRATION

Check for local listing under US Government.

Claims for Social Security retirement, survivors, and disability benefits and Medicare and Supplemental Security Income benefits can be completed by scheduled telephone appointments. Call 1-800-772-1213. The Social Security office will also schedule personal appointments when it is necessary to come into the office. The branch offices provide the same basic function as the district office. Each office administers for the area it serves the retirement, survivors, disability, Supplemental Security Income, and Medicare programs offered under the Social Security protective coverage umbrella.

Social Security Retirement Benefits

Applicants for Social Security retirement benefits must be within three months of being 62 years old. Under certain conditions, children may be eligible for Social Security benefits based on a grandparent's or step-grandparent's or adopted great grandparent's earnings. Generally, a marriage must have lasted at least one year before eligible family members of a retired worker can receive monthly benefits. Benefits can also go to divorced spouses at the age of 62 or older if the marriage lasted 10 years or more. A divorced spouse who has been divorced at least two years can receive benefits at age 62 whether or not his or her former spouse receives them.

Social Security Survivors Benefits

Individuals filing for Social Security Survivors Benefits may start to receive monthly benefits as early as age 60 on the deceased worker's record. If they have a minor child in their care under age 16, they and the child may be eligible for payments at any age. The survivors may be eligible for disability benefits for themselves based on the record of the deceased wage earner at age 50 if their condition is totally disabling. Individuals filing for any type of survivors benefits should bring their own Social Security card, the Social Security card of the deceased worker, their marriage certificate, and (if they have been divorced) a copy of their divorce decree. A notification of death must be sent by the funeral home to the proper Social Security office.

Social Security Disability Program

This program makes monthly payments available to an individual who meets both a work test requirement and the definition of disability. The work test consists of two parts. People aged 31 or over must have worked five full years out of the last 10 years just before the disability occurred. They must have a fully insured status (one calendar quarter of work for each four calendar quarters lapsing since 1950 or the year they attained age 21) for the year in which they became disabled. After 1977, the amount of earnings required per quarter began to increase yearly.

The definition of disability is based on medical evidence provided by the applicant's own doctor or hospital records. In some situations he or she may be asked to have a consultative examination completed and paid for by the state agency that makes disability decisions. Individuals should be prepared to discuss in detail the impairment that causes them to be disabled and why, when it became totally disabling, and how they spend their time at present. They will be asked about the kind of work they have done in the last 15 years; the amount of weight they can reasonably lift; how long they can stand; how doctors, hospitals and clinics have treated them for their disabling impairment and their addresses and telephone numbers; dates they were first seen and periods of confinement in hospitals or clinics; and when they were last seen by the doctor or hospital. An application for any type of disability benefit can be completed by telephone.

Supplemental Security Income Program

The Supplemental Security Income Program (SSI) began in January 1974. It is an income maintenance program providing monthly income to people who are aged 65 or older, blind, or disabled. In some states entitlement to Supplemental Security Income also qualifies recipients for Medicaid and Social Services.

Persons who have little or no regular income and who do not own much property (other than their home) or other things that can be turned into cash such as stocks, bonds, jewelry or other valuables, may get SSI. The aim of the program is to provide monthly cash income to individuals or couples who meet the income and resource limitations.

Medicare Information

Hospital insurance will pay the costs of covered services for the following and follow-up care:

- Up to 90 days of hospital care in a participating hospital during a benefit period. When the patient has been out of the hospital or skilled nursing facility for 60 days in a row (including date of discharge) a new benefit period of 90 days begins.
- Can provide current deductibles up to 100 days of care in participating extended care facility (a skilled nursing home or special part of a hospital which meets the requirements of the law) during each benefit period, provided certain conditions are met.

Medicare can pay for home health visits only if all the following are met:

- Care includes part-time skilled nursing care, physical therapy, or speech therapy; the patient is confined to a home; the physician determines patient needs some health care and sets up a health plan; and the home health agency participates in Medicare.
- Medical insurance will pay 80% of the reasonable charge for various medical services after the deductible, which is subject to change, in each calendar year.

There is a premium for medical insurance that changes yearly. Social Security offices can provide further information on services.

Medicare and Employer Health Plans

Employers with 20 or more employees are required to offer their workers aged 65 or older the same health benefits that are provided to younger workers. They also must offer the spouses aged 65 or older of workers of any age the same health benefits given to younger employees.

For individuals aged 65 or older who continue working and spouses aged 65 or older of a worker who accepts the employer's health plan, Medicare will be the secondary health insurance payer. The employer's health plan will be the primary plan.

For individuals who reject the employer's health plan, Medicare will be the primary health insurance payer and they must file for Medicare supplemental coverage to individuals who reject their health plan.

For individuals under age 65 and disabled, Medicare will be the secondary payer if they choose coverage under their employer's health plan or family member's employer's health plan. This provision applies only to large group health plans that cover employees with at least one employer that has 100 or more workers.

For individuals under age 65, and entitled to Medicare solely on the basis of permanent kidney failure, and who have an employer group health plan, Medicare will be the secondary payer for an initial period of up to 12 months. At the end of the 12-month period, Medicare becomes the primary payer.

Applications for all these benefits may be filed by telephone: 1-800-772-1213.

***Supplementary Security Income (SSI) for Children**
A program through the Social Security office designed to provide a monthly income for families who have a child with a disability that will last more than one year. Application is made through the local Social Security office and is based on diagnosis and family income. The majority of children with a cancer diagnosis are eligible because of their illness, but eligibility will depend on family income.

HOME CARE

*CHILDREN'S HOSPICE INTERNATIONAL

501 Slater's Lane N207, Alexandria, VA 22214
(703) 684-0330

Nonprofit agency that encourages the use of hospices and home care programs for children.

NATIONAL ASSOCIATION FOR HOME CARE

519 C St. NE, Washington, DC 20002
(202) 547-7424

Information and referral to state associations of licensed home health agencies and a membership directory are available from this office. Copies of their pamphlet, "How To Select a Home Care Agency," are available.

NATIONAL HOSPICE ORGANIZATION

1901 N Moore St., Suite 901, Arlington, VA 22209
(703) 243-5900

A nonprofit organization that provides literature and information about hospice to patients and their families and referrals to local, regional, and national resources.

NATIONAL ORGANIZATIONS FOR PATIENT HOUSING

AMERICAN CANCER SOCIETY

The American Cancer Society may help secure hotel/motel accommodations for patients who have to travel long distances for treatment. Contact should be through the local Unit. Some locales may have a special lodge just for housing cancer patients and families. Check with local Unit for this possible resource.

HOUSING AT SPECIFIC CANCER CENTERS

Some treatment centers provide housing or help arrange low-cost housing for patients and families. Check with the specific center for further information.

* RONALD MCDONALD HOUSES

McDonald's Corp., Kroc Drive, Oak Brook, IL 60521
(708) 575-7418

Nonprofit organizations that offer a home away from home for parents and families of children being treated for a serious illness. These can be found in over 60 cities in the United States and Canada and in Sydney, Australia and Paris, France. Each Ronald McDonald House is different, created by a team of concerned local citizens to meet the needs of their own community. Each House is owned and operated by a local not-for-profit organization of volunteers and funded primarily by local contributions. Information regarding the existence of a Ronald McDonald House near a treatment center can be obtained through the social work department of the specific center.

TRANSPORTATION

Air Life Line

1716 X St., Sacramento, CA 95818
(916) 446-0995/FAX (916) 447-5276

This organization is a nonprofit association of over 700 pilots nationwide who donate their time, fuel, and aircraft to fly in medical emergencies. Air Life Line also provides passenger transportation for medical purposes. In addition to flying patients for cancer treatment, they also fly terminally ill patients home from medical centers and family members to hospitals to see their loved ones while they undergo lengthy medical treatment. A patient requiring air transportation can be flown a distance of 500 miles one way. Criteria for acceptance include: financial need, an ambulatory patient, a signed physician's statement verifying stable health, and the ability to travel in a small-engine plane.

American Medical Support Flight Team (AMSFT)

2452 Brookhurst Dr., Atlanta, GA 30338
(404) 458-0674
5524 Meander Lane, Lake Wales, FL 33853
(813) 439-3780

AMSFT is a nonprofit volunteer pilot association and community service organization that provides free air transportation in private aircraft to health care agencies, blood banks, donor organ banks, and needy individuals with health care problems. A family member may fly as well. Patients must be mobile and medically stable. Most flights need to be within a 500-mile radius of the plane's home base.

Angel Flight

3237 Donald Douglas Loop S, Santa Monica, CA 90405
(213) 390-2958

Angel Flight is a nonprofit volunteer pilot association and community service organization that provides free air transportation in private aircraft to health care agencies, blood banks, donor organ banks, and needy individuals with health care problems. A family member may fly as well. Patients must be mobile and medically stable. Most flights need to be within a 500-mile radius of the plane's home base.

CANCER INFORMATION SERVICE

1-800-422-6237

Provides listing of air transport services specific to caller's geographic area.

CORPORATE ANGEL NETWORK, INC.

Westchester County Airport , Building 1, White Plains, NY 10604

A nonprofit organization designed to give cancer patients who require transportation anywhere in the United States the use of available seats on corporate aircraft. Patients must be ambulatory and not require any specific equipment or services enroute. They must have proper medical authorization for the flight, either to a center for specialized treatment or to their home. Local ground transportation is handeled by patients' families or local volunteers, not by the participating corporation. There is no financial need criteria. Referrals will be accepted from social service and medical personnel, family members, or friends; a Corporate Angel Network representative must speak directly to the patient or the person traveling with the patient in order to explain the program thoroughly. Requests for transportation will be taken when a definite travel date is known.

MERCY MEDICAL AIRLIFT (MMA)

P.O. Box 1940, Manassas, VA 22110

(703) 361-1191/24-hour access service : (202) 389-0024

A nonprofit charitable organization dedicated to alleviating suffering, hardship, and family crisis through the provision of medical air transportation for patients who cannot afford the cost of commercial air ambulance. Patients and families are served regardless of race, sex, religion, age, or national origin.

MMA serves the 14 states in the mid-Atlantic and Northeastern regions of the country. Patients will be picked up from within this area and taken elsewhere in the country or they will be picked up elsewhere and brought back into this region.

MMA will advise and/or assist families needing any form of medical air transportation. In cases where transport by commercial airlines is feasible, MMA will provide a volunteer transport nurse to accompany the patient and family member.

*WISH ORGANIZATIONS

The wish organizations listed below are all voluntary organizations dedicated to providing a wish for children up to the age of 18 with life-threatening illnesses. The addresses listed are all national addresses but these offices can provide contact people for local areas.

*THE CANDLELIGHTERS CHILDHOOD CANCER FOUNDATION

1312 18th St. NW, Suite 200, Washington, DC 20036
1-800-366-2223

Candlelighters has a roster of wish fulfillment organizations that grant wishes for children with life-threatening, chronic, or terminal illnesses.

DISNEY WORLD VISITS

1-800-457-1976

* MAKE-A-WISH FOUNDATION OF AMERICA

2600 North Central Ave., Suite 936, Phoenix, AZ 85004
1-800-722-9474
(602) 240-6600

SUNSHINE FOUNDATION

4010 Levick St., Philadelphia, PA 19135
(215) 335-2622

PROFESSIONAL ORGANIZATIONS

AMERICAN ASSOCIATION OF CANCER EDUCATION (AACE)

University of Alabama-Birmingham
(Michael Brooks, MD)
Birmingham, AL 35292
(205) 934-3054

A multidisciplinary organization that provides education and training programs for professionals involved in cancer care. Annual meetings are held and members receive the AACE *Handbook* upon joining.

AMERICAN SOCIETY OF CLINICAL ONCOLOGY

435 N Michigan Ave., Suite 1717, Chicago, IL 60611
(312) 644-0828

Promotes and fosters the exchange of information relating to neoplastic diseases with particular emphasis on human biology, diagnosis, treatment, and psychosocial impact of disease.

*ASSOCIATION OF PEDIATRIC ONCOLOGY SOCIAL WORKERS (APOSW)

An international association for pediatric oncology social workers that provides networking and support. APOSW publishes a quarterly newsletter, sponsors an annual conference, and offers a reduced membership rate to NAOSW members. For current membership chairperson, call the American Cancer Society, (404) 320-3333.

NATIONAL ASSOCIATION OF ONCOLOGY SOCIAL WORKERS

1275 York Ave., MRI 1009, New York, NY 10021
(212) 639-7015

The National Association of Oncology Social Workers (NAOSW) is a national organization for professional social workers in oncology. It was created in 1983 by social workers interested in oncology and existing national cancer organizations. Its functions include advocating sound public and professional programs and policies for cancer patients and providing valuable services to its members.

NAOSW members receive support from individuals working in similar areas through the organization's network; a quarterly newsletter filled with timely and up-to-date news on clinical, educational, and research activities of colleagues, relevant public issues, and meeting announcements; career opportunities; discounts on the NAOSW annual meeting that provides state-of-the-art presentations, panels, and workshops and technical assistance in clinical, academic, and administrative areas; and leadership voting privileges.

NAOSW offers members of the Association of Pediatric Oncology Social Workers all the NAOSW membership benefits, plus a reduced membership rate.

EDUCATION AND TRAINING

Many comprehensive cancer treatment centers and other cancer-related hospitals and agencies offer special training in oncology. Contact the American Cancer Society or NAOSW for specific information.

AMERICAN CANCER SOCIETY TRAINING GRANTS IN CLINICAL ONCOLOGY SOCIAL WORK

The American Cancer Society annually awards Clinical Oncology Social Work training grants to qualifying hospitals and medical centers that train clinical oncology social workers to provide cancer patients and their families with psychosocial services. Grants are available to second-year students in master's programs and post-master's social workers within five years of graduation. The master's training introduces social workers to the special needs of cancer patients and their families. The post-master's training helps prepare candidates for advanced clinical practice and research related to psychosocial needs of cancer patients and their families. Both programs prepare candidates for direct clinical practice with cancer patients and their families. A maximum of four applications are considered for each institution–master's and post-master's training in pediatric and adult practice settings. An institution is eligible to receive only one award.

Contact the Clinical Awards Program, American Cancer Society, National Office, 1599 Clifton Road NE, Atlanta, GA 30329, (404) 320-3333.

NAOSW STANDARDS OF PRACTICE IN ONCOLOGY SOCIAL WORK†

INTRODUCTION

Oncology social work is the professional discipline that provides social work services to patients, families and significant others facing the impact of a potential or actual diagnosis of cancer. The scope of oncology social work includes clinical practice, education, administration and research. The standards of practice provided in this document are intended for clinical social workers practicing in the specialty of oncology social work.

The Masters in Social Work degree provides oncology social workers with theoretical knowledge, clinical expertise and practical experience with patients. In addition, oncology social workers often receive specialized training in cancer care through continuing education, inservice training and on-the-job experience. They are responsible for the provision of counseling and linkage to community services for cancer patients and their families across the full cancer-continuum, including prevention, survivorship, chronic or terminal care and bereavement.

Oncology social workers facilitate patients' adjustment to illness and the maintenance of optimal individual and family functioning. Services are designed to promote the patient's best utilization of the health care system, the optimal development of coping strategies and the mobilization of community resources to support maximum functioning.

Oncology social workers offer individual and group social services, engage in supportive counseling with families and advocate for the needs of patients. They provide case management, linking patients with

† *Long Range Planning Committee of NAOSW, Lois Weinstein, CSW, chairperson. NAOSW: 1275 York Ave., MR1107, New York, NY 10021, (212) 639-7015.*

the variety of services necessary to meet the person's multiple needs. They function collaboratively with other cancer care professionals in treatment planning for patients as well as in discharge planning when care is being provided within institutions.

Oncology social workers are found in a wide range of settings ranging from private practice to community-based agencies to specialty cancer centers. The great majority have a specialty practice within a general hospital setting.

STANDARDS OF PRACTICE

STANDARD I. QUALIFICATIONS

Oncology social workers shall be knowledgeable about oncological diseases and their treatments, psychosocial implications for individuals and families, appropriate interventions and available community and governmental resources. Oncology social workers must have knowledge of the usual course of cancer and its treatment so that patients and families can be helped to anticipate and deal with changes in family life.

The oncology social worker shall be masters prepared from a graduate program accredited by the Council on Social Work Education. It is preferred that the graduate have had prior employment or field placement experience in a health care setting.

STANDARD II. SERVICES TO PATIENTS AND FAMILIES

Oncology social work programs shall provide the following clinical and programmatic services:

A. Completion of a psychosocial assessment of the patient and family's response to the cancer diagnosis to include:
   1. stages in human development;
   2. knowledge about cancer and its treatment including level of understanding, reactions, and expectations;
   3. patient and family psychosocial functioning including strengths, coping skills and supports;
   4. characteristics of the patient's family and/or social group;
   5. the source, availability, and adequacy of community resources.

B. Development of a case plan with patient and family based on mutually agreed upon goals to enhance, maintain and promote optimal psychosocial functioning through cancer treatment and its outcome.

C. Utilization of appropriate clinical intervention designed to address current and/or future problems as the patient's medical and psychosocial needs evolve.

D. Establishment of screening criteria for case finding and outreach activities.

E. Development of knowledge of cancer and its treatment and knowledge of current trends.

F. Maintenance of knowledge of community resources and governmental programs available from local and national health and welfare agencies including expertise in accessing these for patients and families.

G. Organization and facilitation of patient and family education in and outside the organization.

H. Advocacy for and protection of patients' dignity, confidentiality, rights, and access to care within and outside the organization.

I. Development of knowledge of research findings that relate to or evaluate the effectiveness of practice.

Standard III. Services to Organizations

Oncology social work programs shall address organizational needs including the following:

A. Provision of consultation to other disciplines and staff regarding biopsychosocial, environmental and cultural factors that affect oncology care.

B. Collaboration with other disciplines and staff in the areas of comprehensive patient and family care, research and psychosocial education.

C. Support services designed to address staff management of the stresses inherent in oncologic practice.

D. Compliance with recording required by the organization, provision of statistical information on activities, and review of activities with an aim of improving services, insuring quality and developing programs.

STANDARD IV. SERVICES TO THE COMMUNITY

Oncology social work programs shall address community needs including the following:

A. Identification of unmet needs and underserved groups.

B. Provision of services to at-risk populations.

C. Consultation and collaboration with outside organizations and professionals to promote health, to educate the community at large, and to develop programs to better serve the community.

D. Liaison between the organization and the community, and coordination of activities.

STANDARD V. COLLABORATION

Oncology social workers, as members of a health care team, shall collaborate with other professional disciplines in the planning and provision of services to cancer patients.

STANDARD VI. DOCUMENTATION

Oncology social work entries in the patient's case record shall be clearly and concisely written permitting ongoing communication with other professionals involved in planning the patient's care. Documentation should conform to agency standards and insure accountability and confidentiality.

STANDARD VII. PROFESSIONAL DEVELOPMENT

The personal and professional development of the oncology social worker shall be realized by a defined program of continuing education to supplement and encourage the ongoing development of clinical, educational and research skills. Oncology social work staff shall be provided with appropriate orientation, supervision, continuing education, training programs and regular evaluations. Supervision/consultation shall be provided by a senior social worker experienced in oncology social work.

GLOSSARY

This "glossary" defines some of the medical and scientific terms commonly used by physicians, nurses, researchers, and technicians who deal with cancer on a daily basis. (Reprinted with permission of the American Cancer Society.)

A

Adenocarcinoma–A form of cancer that involves the cells lining the walls of many different organs in the body.

Adjuvant Treatment–Treatment that is added to increase effectiveness of a primary therapy. In cancer, adjuvant treatment usually refers to chemotherapy or radiotherapy administered after surgery to increase the likelihood of cure.

Androgen–A male sex hormone. Androgens may be used in patients with breast cancer to treat recurrence of the disease.

Antibiotic–A substance derived from a mold or bacteria that can be used to treat diseases. Penicillin is the most familiar type used to treat infection. Certain special antibiotics are effective drugs in cancer chemotherapy.

Antibody–A protein in the blood that fights against an invading foreign agent (antigen). Each antibody works against a particular antigen.

Antigen–A foreign agent that stimulates the formation of antibodies in the body.

Antimetabolites–Anticancer drugs that interfere with the processes of DNA production, and thus prevent cell division.

Asymptomatic–Without obvious signs or symptoms of disease. Cancer may cause symptoms or warning signs, but, especially in its early stages, cancer may develop and grow without producing symptoms. Cancer detection tests attempt to discover it at an early, asymptomatic stage when the chances for cure are highest. (See **Screening**.)

Atypical–Not usual; abnormal. For example, cancer is the result of atypical cell division.

Axilla–The armpit. Lymph glands in the armpit are called the axillary nodes. Certain cancers, such as breast cancer, spread to the axillary nodes. Axillary lymph nodes are usually removed by surgery to determine if breast cancer is present and if treatment with chemotherapy is necessary.

B

Barium Enema–Use of barium sulfate introduced into the intestinal tract by an enema to allow x-ray exam of the large bowel.

Basal Cell Carcinoma–The most common form of skin cancer. Basal carcinoma grows slowly and seldom spreads to other areas of the body. It is easily detected and cured when treated promptly.

Benign Tumor–An abnormal growth that is not cancer and does not spread to other areas of the body.

Bilateral–Pertaining to both sides of the body. For example, bilateral breast cancer.

Biological Response Modifiers–A new class of compounds produced in the body, such as interferon, that fight cancer by stimulating the body's immune system.

Biopsy–The surgical removal of a small piece of tissue for microscopic examination to determine if cancer cells are present. Biopsy is the most important procedure in diagnosing cancer.

Blood Count–Examination of a blood specimen in which the number of white blood cells, red blood cells, and platelets are determined. For example, in patients with leukemia the blood count may show an abnormally high number of white blood cells.

Bone Marrow–The soft, fatty substance filling the cavities of bones. Blood cells are manufactured in bone marrow. The bone marrow is sampled in leukemia, lymphoma, multiple myeloma, and other cancers affecting blood cells to determine the diagnosis and response to treatment.

Bone Marrow Biopsy and Aspiration–A procedure in which a needle is inserted into the center of a bone, usually the hip or breast bone, to remove a small amount of bone marrow for microscopic examination.

Brain Scan–A technique in which radioactive dye is injected into a vein, so that images of the brain can be recorded. Brain scans may be used for the detection of cancers starting in brain tissue or from other areas of the body.

Breast Self-Exam (BSE)–A simple procedure to examine breasts thoroughly; recommended once a month for all women to do themselves between regular physician checkups.

C

Cancer–A general term for a large group of diseases (more than 100), all characterized by uncontrolled growth and spread of abnormal cells. Cancer cells are abnormal and eventually form tumors that invade and destroy surrounding tissue; they may even spread via the lymph system or bloodstream to distant areas of the body. (See **Metastasis** and **Malignant Tumor**.)

Cancer Cell–A cell that divides and reproduces abnormally.

Cancer-Related Checkup–Periodic health examination for cancer in asymptomatic persons (without obvious signs or symptoms) in order to detect the disease at an early, curable stage.

Carcinogens–Any substance that initiates or promotes the development of cancer. For example, asbestos is a proven carcinogen.

Carcinoma–A form of cancer that develops in tissues covering or lining organs of the body, such as the skin, the uterus, the lung, or the breast.

Carcinoma in Situ–An early stage in development, when the cancer is still confined to the tissues of origin. In situ carcinomas are highly curable.

Cell–The basic structural unit of life. All living matter is composed of cells.

Cervix–Any "necklike" structure; usually refers to the neck of the uterus where cancer may occur.

Chemoprevention–In cancer, this term is used to describe attempts at prevention of disease by drugs, chemicals, vitamins and/or minerals. The concept is under study but is not yet ready for wide application.

Chemotherapy–Treatment of disease, such as cancer, by drugs.

Clinical Trial–The scientific evaluation of the means to prevent, detect, diagnose, or treat disease in human beings. Clinical trials are conducted after experiments in animals have shown evidence of potential effectiveness and preliminary studies in humans suggest usefulness.

Colon–The part of the large intestine that extends from the end of the small intestine to the rectum.

Colonoscopy–A technique used to visually examine the entire colon by means of a lighted, flexible instrument, called a fiberoptic colonoscope. This procedure may also obtain biopsy specimens of suspicious tissue.

Colostomy–A surgical procedure that creates an artificial opening in the abdominal wall for elimination of body wastes from the colon. It can be either temporary or permanent. Most colon cancers do not require colostomies if they are found early and treated promptly.

Combination Chemotherapy–Treatment consisting of the use of two or more chemicals to achieve the most effective results.

Combined Modality Therapy–Two or more types of treatment–surgery, radiation therapy, chemotherapy, or immunotherapy–used alternatively or together for maximum effectiveness. For example, surgery for cancer is often followed by chemotherapy to destroy any random cancer cells that may have spread from the original site.

Computerized Tomography Scans–Commonly called CT scans, these specialized x-ray studies can find cancer or metastases. CT scans have revolutionized the diagnosis of cancer and other diseases.

Cyst–An abnormal saclike structure that contains liquid or semisolid material; may be benign or malignant. Lumps in the breast are often found to be harmless cysts and not cancer.

Cytology–Study of cells under a microscope. Cells that have been sloughed off or scraped off organs such as the uterus, lungs, bladder, or stomach are microscopically examined for signs of cancer. Also called exfoliative cytology. (See **Pap Test**.)

D

Detection–The discovery of an abnormality in an asymptomatic or symptomatic person. "Early Detection" is the discovery of an abnormality by health professionals through a special effort designed to screen for asymptomatic disease, or by people themselves who have been made alert to the existence of signs or symptoms.

Diagnosis–The process of identifying a disease by its characteristic signs, symptoms, and laboratory findings. In patients with cancer, the earlier the diagnosis is made, the better the chance for cure.

Digital Rectal Exam–A procedure in which the physician inserts a finger into the rectum to examine this area (as well as the prostate gland in men) for signs of cancer.

DNA–One of two nucleic acids (the other is RNA) found in the nucleus of all cells. DNA contains genetic information on cell growth, division, and function.

E

Endometrium–The inner mucous membrane that forms the uterine wall. Endometrial cancer generally affects women between 50 and 64 years old.

Endoscopy–Any procedure that uses a hollow tubelike instrument to visualize and biopsy otherwise inaccessible areas of the body such as the esophagus, stomach, colon, bladder, or lung.

Enterostomal Therapist–A health professional trained to assist patients in the proper care of stomas–openings in the abdominal wall created to remove wastes.

Epidemiology–Study of disease incidence and distribution in populations, as well as the relationship between environment and disease. Cancer epidemiology studies how physical surroundings, occupational hazards, and personal habits (smoking, diet, and life-style) may contribute to the development of cancer.

Erythroplasia–Red lesions, grainy or smooth, on the mucous membranes of the mouth, that may indicate an early cancer.

Esophageal Speech–An acquired technique of speaking used by larngectomees who have had their voice boxes removed. Air is expelled from the esophagus, thus vibrating the walls of the pharynx and esophagus to produce sound.

Estrogen–A female hormone secreted by the ovaries, which is essential for menstruation, reproduction, and the development of secondary sex characteristics such as breasts. Some patients with breast cancer are given estrogen to inhibit tumor growth.

Etiology–Study of the causes of disease. In cancer, there are probably multiple etiologies.

F

Five-Year Survival–A term commonly used as the statistical basis for successful treatment. A patient with cancer is generally considered cured after five or more years without recurrence of disease.

Frozen Section–A technique in which tissue is removed by biopsy, then frozen, cut into thin slices, stained, and examined under a microscope. A pathologist can rapidly examine a frozen section for immediate diagnosis. This procedure is often done during surgery to help the physician decide the most appropriate course of action.

Genes–Located in the nucleus of the cell, genes contain hereditary information that is transferred from cell to cell. A process called genetic engineering may be used eventually to modify heredity and correct impaired immunity.

H

High Risk–When the chance of developing cancer is greater than normally seen in the general population. Patients may be at high risk from many factors including heredity (e.g., a family history of breast cancer), personal habits (e.g., smoking), or the environment (e.g., overexposure to sunlight). (See **Risk Factor.**)

Hodgkin's Disease–A form of cancer that affects the lymph system. Hodgkin's disease generally occurs in adults and can now be successfully treated in the majority of patients.

Hormone–Secreted by various organs in the body, hormones help regulate growth, metabolism, and reproduction. Some hormones are used as treatment following surgery for breast, ovarian, and prostate cancers.

Hospice–A concept of psychosocial and supportive care to meet the special needs of patients and their families during the terminal stages of illness. The care is provided both in outpatient and inpatient settings.

Hysterectomy–The surgical removal of the uterus. May be combined with removal of the ovaries (oophorectomy).

I

Immunology–Study of the body's mechanisms of resistance against disease or invasion by foreign substances.

Immunotherapy–A treatment that stimulates the body's own defense mechanisms to combat disease, such as cancer.

In Situ–In place; localized and confined to one area. A very early stage of cancer.

Incidence–The extent to which disease occurs in the population. Cancer incidence is the estimated number of new cases of cancer diagnosed each year.

Interferon–A natural body protein produced by normal cells that is capable of killing cancer cells or stopping their unrestrained growth. Interferon was originally discovered as an antiviral agent, but has now been found to have some anticancer activity as well. Interferon may be artificially produced in large quantities using the technique of recombinant DNA.
Involuntary Smoking–When nonsmokers breathe cigarette smoke from other people, they are involuntarily smoking. The risk of lung cancer in nonsmokers is now being studied. Also called passive smoking, side-stream smoking, and second-hand smoking.

L

Laryngectomy–The surgical removal of the larynx or voice box, resulting in the loss of normal speech. A laryngectomee is someone who has undergone this operation. (See **Esophageal Speech.**)
Leukemia–Cancer of the blood-forming tissues (bone marrow, lymph nodes, spleen). Leukemia is characterized by the overproduction of abnormal, immature white blood cells.
Leukoplakia–White plaques on the mucous membranes of the mouth and gums; may be precancerous.
Localized Cancer–A cancer still confined to its site of origin.
Lymph–A clear fluid circulating throughout the body (in the lymphatic system) that contains white blood cells and antibodies.
Lymph Gland–Also called lymph node. These glands produce lymph. They normally act as filters of impurities in the body.

M

Malignant Tumor–A mass of cancer cells. A malignant tumor may invade surrounding tissues or spread to distant areas of the body. (See **Metastasis**.)
Mammogram–The image produced by a low-dose x-ray of the breast.
Mammography– A screening and diagnostic technique that uses low-dose x-rays to find tumors in the breast. Mammography can reveal a tumor too small to be felt even by the most experienced physician. The procedure may be used as a detection test in all women of the appropriate age group who do not have symptoms. All suspicious breast lumps must be biopsied to determine whether or not they are cancer.
Melanoma–A type of skin cancer. While most skin cancers rarely

spread to other areas of the body and are easily treated and cured, melanoma can be more aggressive if not detected early.

Metastasis–The spread of cancer cells to distant areas of the body by way of the lymph system or bloodstream. The term "metastases" refers to these new cancer sites.

Mitosis–The process of cell reproduction.

Monoclonal Antibodies–Antibodies designed to seek out chosen targets on cancer cells. They are under study to deliver chemotherapy and radiotherapy directly to a cancer, thus killing the cancer cell and sparing healthy tissue. Studies are also under way to determine if monoclonal antibodies can be produced to detect and diagnose cancer cells at a very early, curable stage.

Morbidity–Sickness. The term usually refers to the proportion of people with an illness.

Mortality–Mortality rates reflect the number of deaths in a given population.

N

Neoplasm–Any new abnormal growth. Neoplasms may be benign or malignant, but the term is generally used to describe a cancer.

Nodule–A small solid mass.

Oncogene–Certain stretches of cellular DNA, genes that when inappropriately activated contribute to the malignant transformation of a cell.

Oncologist–A physician who specializes in cancer treatment, after undergoing extensive training and examinations.

Oncology–The science dealing with the physical, chemical, and biologic properties and features of cancer, including causes and the disease process.

P

Palliative Treatment–Therapy that relieves symptoms, such as pain, but does not alter the course of disease. Its primary purpose is to improve the quality of life.

Palpation–A procedure using the hands to examine organs such as the breast or prostate. A palpable mass is one that can be felt.

Pap Test–Developed by the late Dr. George Papanicolaou, it is a simple microscopic examination of cells. This test can detect cancer of the cervix at an early, highly curable stage. (See **Cytology.**)
Pathology–Study of disease through the microscopic examination of body tissues and organs. Any tumor suspected of being cancerous must be diagnosed by pathologic examination.
Pelvic Examination–A manual internal examination of the female reproductive organs, through the vagina and rectum.
Placebo– An inert substance, such as a sugar pill. A placebo may be used in clinical trials to compare the effects of a given treatment against no treatment.
Platelet–A substance found in the blood that is necessary for blood clotting. Platelet transfusions are used in cancer patients to prevent or control bleeding when the number of platelets has decreased.
Polyp–A nodular growth of tissue developing in the lining of a cavity such as the colon, the nose, or the vocal cords. Polyps may be benign or malignant.
Precancerous–Abnormal cellular changes that are potentially capable of becoming cancer. These early lesions are very amenable to treatment and cure. Also called premalignant.
Prevalence–The number of patients with a disease in the population at a specific time. For example, the prevalence of esophageal cancer is higher in blacks than whites.
Prevention–The reduction of cancer by eliminating or reducing contact with carcinogenic agents. A change in life-style such as not smoking, for example, can prevent lung and many other cancers.
Procto–An abbreviation for sigmoidoscopy. An examination of the rectum and lower colon with a hollow lighted tube called a sigmoidoscope. A procto is used to detect colorectal polyps and cancer.
Prognosis–A prediction of the course of disease; the future prospects for the patient. For example, breast cancer patients who receive treatment early have a good prognosis.
Prostate–A gland located at the base of the bladder in males.
Prosthesis–An artificial replacement for a missing part of the body such as a breast or limb.

R

Radioactive Implant–A source of high-dose radiation that is placed directly into and around a cancer to kill the cancer cells.

Radiotherapist–A physician with special training in the use of x-ray energy for the treatment of cancer.

Radiotherapy–Treatment of cancer with high-energy radiation. Radiation therapy may be used to reduce the size of a cancer before surgery, or to destroy any remaining cancer cells after surgery. Radiotherapy can be helpful in shrinking recurrent cancers to relieve symptoms.

Rectum–The last five to six inches of the colon leading to the anus.

Recurrence (Local)–Reappearance of cancer at its original site after a period of remission.

Regional Involvement–The spread of cancer from its original site to nearby surrounding areas. Regional cancers are confined to one location in the body.

Rehabilitation–Programs that help patients adjust and return to a full productive life. Rehabilitation may involve physical restoration, such as the use of prostheses, and counseling and emotional support. (See **Prosthesis**.)

Relapse–The reappearance of cancer after a disease-free period.

Remission–Complete or partial disappearance of the signs and symptoms of disease in response to treatment. The period during which a disease is under control. A remission, however, is not necessarily a cure.

Risk Factor–Anything that increases an individual's chance of getting a disease, such as cancer. For example, the major risk factor for skin cancer is overexposure to the sun.

Risk Reduction–Those techniques used to reduce the chances of developing cancer. For example, low-fat diets may help reduce the risk of breast cancer.

S

Sarcoma–A form of cancer that arises in the supportive tissues, such as bone, cartilage, fat, or muscle.

Secondary Tumor–A tumor that develops as a result of metastases or spread beyond the original cancer.

Screening–The search for disease, such as cancer, in individuals without known symptoms. Screening may refer to coordinated mass programs in large populations.

Side Effects–Usually describes after effects or secondary effects of treatment. For example, hair loss may be a side effect of chemotherapy; nausea may be the side effect of radiation therapy or chemotherapy.
Sigmoidoscopy–The visual inspection of the rectum and lower colon by a tubular instrument called a sigmoidoscope passed through the rectum. The instrument may be either a rigid or flexible instrument. (See **Procto**.)
Squamous Cell Carcinoma–A form of skin cancer that usually appears as red, scaly patches or nodules typically on lips, face, tips of ears. It can spread to other parts of the body if untreated.
Staging–An evaluation of the extent of disease, such as cancer. A classification based on stage at diagnosis helps determine appropriate treatment and prognosis.
Stoma–A surgically created opening. For example, a stoma is made in the abdominal wall for elimination of wastes when the colon and/or rectum can no longer perform this function. (See **Colostomy**.)
Stool Blood Test–A simple chemical test to detect invisible (occult) blood in the feces. It is used to detect early signs of gastrointestinal conditions including polyps and cancers of the colon and rectum.
Surgery–A procedure to remove a part of the body or to find out if disease is present.

T

Testes (Testicles)–The two male sex organs suspended in a pouch, called the scrotum, below the penis.
Testicular Self-Examination (TSE)–A simple manual examination of the testes. Should be performed monthly.
Tissue–A collection of similar cells. There are four basic types of tissues in the body: epithelial, connective, muscle, and nerve.
Tumor–An abnormal tissue swelling or mass; may be either benign or malignant.

U

Ultrasound Examination–The use of high-frequency sound waves to locate a tumor deep inside the body. Also called ultrasonography.
Unproven Methods of Cancer Management–Scientifically untested methods of preventing, diagnosing, or treating cancer. The American Cancer Society maintains an extensive reference file on unproven methods of cancer management; information is available on request.

Uterus–A female reproductive organ; the womb in which an unborn child develops until birth.

V

Vaccine–A substance injected into the body to stimulate resistance to a specific disease.
Vagina–A female reproductive organ. Also called the birth canal.
Virus–Tiny living organisms that invade cells, alter the cells' chemistry, and cause them to produce more viruses. Viruses are the cause of many diseases. In animals, several viruses have been shown to produce cancer. Their role in the development of cancer in man is now being studied.

W

Warning Signals–Signs or symptoms that suggest the presence of cancer. The American Cancer Society urges individuals to contact their physicians if they have one of cancer's warning signals.

X-ray–Radiant energy used to diagnose and treat disease, such as cancer. High doses of x-rays can kill cancer cells.

BILL OF RIGHTS†

FOR CANCER PATIENTS

I have the right to be told the truth about my disease.

I have the right to feel bad if I receive bad news.

I have the right to talk to my doctor and my family about cancer. And, I have the right to privacy in refusing to talk with others about it if that is my choice.

I have the right to be treated as a person and not merely as a "patient" while I am sick. The fact that I am sick does not give others the right to make decisions for me.

I have the right to think about other things besides my cancer. I do not have to allow cancer to control every detail of my life.

I have the right to ask others for help in the things I cannot do for myself, within reason.

I always have the right to hope–for a full cure, a longer life, or a happier life here and now.

I have the right and it is OK to be angry with people I love. My anger does not mean I have stopped loving them.

I have the right to cope with my cancer in my own way, and my family has the right to cope with it in theirs. Our ways may be different, but that is OK.

I have the right to be free of pain if that is my choice.

---

† *Reprinted with permission of Cancer Family Care, 7162 Reading Road, Suite 1050, Cincinnati, Ohio 45237-3833.*

FOR FAMILY MEMBERS

I have the right to enjoy my own good health without feeling guilty. It is not my fault that someone I love has cancer.

I have the right to choose whom I will talk to about cancer. If I hurt others' feelings because they are asking too many questions, it is not my fault.

I have the right to know what is going on in our family, even if I am a child. I have the right to be told the truth about the cancer in words I can understand.

I have the right to disagree with the patient even if he or she has cancer. I can feel angry with someone and not always feel guilty, because sickness does not stop someone from being a real person.

I have the right to feel what I feel now, not what someone else says I "should" feel.

I have the right to look after my own needs, even if they do not seem as great as the patient's. I am permitted to take "time out" from the cancer without feeling disloyal.

I have the right to get outside help for the patient if I cannot manage all the responsibilities of home care myself.

I have the right to get help for myself, even if others in my family choose not to get help.

INDEX

CONTRIBUTORS

Diane Blum, MSW, ACSW, is executive director of Cancer Care, New York, New York.

David B. Callan, MSW, is clinical supervisor for Cancer Family Care, Inc. in Cincinnati, Ohio.

Grace Christ, DSW, CSW, ACSW, is on the faculty of the Columbia University School of Social Work, New York, New York.

Nancy F. Cincotta, MSW, CSW, ACSW, CCLS, is preceptor of the social work department at The Mount Sinai Medical Center, New York, New York.

Catherine S. Cordoba, MSW, ACSW, is retired and lives in San Francisco, California.

Sue Cooper, MSW, CSW-ACP, is a consultant in AIDS-related health policy and education and is based in Houston, Texas.

Paula R. Fogelberg, MSW, LCSW, is in private practice in Franklin, Tennessee.

Patricia Fobair, MSW, MPH, LCSW, is affiliated with the Stanford University Hospital Department of Radiation Oncology, Stanford University Medical Center, Stanford, California.

Julia H. Gaskell, MSW, MPH, is former clinical social worker at Duke University Medical Center, Durham, North Carolina. She lives in Chapel Hill, North Carolina.

Joan Hermann, MSW, ACSW, is director of the social work services department at Fox Chase Cancer Center, Philadelphia, Pennsylvania.

Marie Lauria, MSW, ACSW, is clinical social worker/supervisor, University of North Carolina Hospitals, and clinical associate professor in pediatrics, University of North Carolina School of Medicine, Chapel Hill, North Carolina.

Philip A. Pizzo, MD, is affiliated with the pediatric branch of the National Cancer Institute, Bethesda, Maryland.

David S. Rosenthal, MD, is director of Harvard University Health Services, Cambridge, Massachusetts.

Judith W. Ross, MSW, ACSW, LISW, is director of social work for MetroHealth Systems, Cleveland, Ohio, and editor-in-chief of *Health* and *Social Work.*

Naomi M. Stearns, MSW, LICSW, is director of social work at Dana-Farber Cancer Institute, Boston, Massachusetts.

Allison Stovall, MSW, CSW-ACP, is affiliated with the University of Texas MD Anderson Cancer Center, Houston, Texas.